| ADVANCE PRAISE FOR |

ONE BOWL

"Don's book offers a rare gift to the reader—it unlocks a passage-way in your mind that opens your understanding to a new creative direction to choose on your journey with food. *One Bowl* will nourish your courage to be at one with yourself."

—MARY HARPER, Ph.D., Founding Director, Center for Changing Systems

"Inspired! Not just another 'diet book,' *One Bowl* provides a sensible and easy-to-follow formula for rethinking one's relationship with food. Well-written and entertaining, it's a must for anyone interested in leading a healthier life."

—PAUL L. SANDBERG, entertainment lawyer and film producer

"What an eye opener—after one quick reading I have slowed down—no more eating over the sink or while paying the bills. I had my first meal alone and loved it. I got to taste the food instead of trying to create conversation."

—GRETA ROSS, events planner and catering consultant

"A real eye-opener. *One Bowl* isn't about diets, or nutritional supplements, or pre-packaged food. It's a fundamentally different way of thinking about food. I know that it works because I've seen it in action. Don Gerrard is twenty years younger than I am, and he's at least twice as healthy. With this book, I finally know his secret. I'm already putting this to work in my own life."

—JEFF EDWARDS, author of *Dome City Blues*

"In a time where there appears to be no limits to anything, Don Gerrard shows that there is art and satisfaction in the practice of restraint."

—STANLEY KELEMAN, author of *Living Your Dying* and *Emotional Anatomy*

| DON GERRARD |

ONE BOWL

DON GERRARD is a writer, editor, and publisher with over forty years experience in the book business. He's had a lifelong interest in health-related subjects, including homeopathy and food awareness. Gerrard lives in Tucson, Arizona.

| MARLOWE & COMPANY |

ONE BOWL

ONE BOWL

A GUIDE TO
EATING FOR
BODY
AND
SPIRIT

■

MARLOWE & COMPANY | NEW YORK

ONE BOWL: *A Guide to Eating for Body and Spirit*

Copyright © 1974, 2001 by Don Gerrard

Published by
Marlowe & Company
An Imprint of Avalon Publishing Group Incorporated
161 William St., 16th Floor
New York, NY 10038

LIBRARY OF CONGRESS CATALOGING-IN-PUBLICATION DATA
Gerrard, Don.
One bowl: a guide to eating for body and spirit / by Don Gerrard.
p. cm.
ISBN 1-56924-627-0
1. Weight loss. 2. Hunger. 3. Food habits. I. Title.
RM222.2 .G47 2001
613.2'5—dc21
00-048944

9 8 7 6 5 4 3 2 1

Designed by Pauline Neuwirth, Neuwirth & Associates, Inc.

Printed in the United States of America
Distributed by Publishers Group West

AUTHOR'S NOTE: Our language has no singular ungendered pronoun
forms. In order to avoid writing the clumsy expressions *he or she*, *him or her*
throughout the book, I have adopted *they*, *them*, and *their*
wherever the singular pronoun should be used.

This book is dedicated to three important people in my life:

Eugenia Rush Gerrard, my extraordinary wife,
who pointed out many years ago that I needed
to lose some weight, thereby setting this journey
of greater food awareness into motion.

Anne Kent Rush, my very creative friend,
who helped me with this book more than
she realizes. Kent showed me the
spiritual dimension of my quest.

Hal Zina Bennett, my excellent editor, without
whose faithful vision this new edition would
not have been possible.

I owe all three of you for many years of friendship.
You have made my journey worthwhile!

CONTENTS

CONTENTS

CONTENTS

CONTENTS

CONTENTS

CONTENTS

ONE BOWL

IS THIS BOOK FOR YOU?

I pay close attention to the sensation of hunger in my body, the opening note of what soon becomes a whole symphony of inner sensations associated with my natural digestive processes. When I sit down to eat a meal, this symphony of inner sensations begins, and it continues as long as I'm eating. It is literally the background music of my body's life.

I wrote this small book as a way to share with you my insights about eating. The One Bowl method that I will describe in these pages first began as a way to lose weight but very quickly became a whole new way of looking at my total relationship to food and eating. The One Bowl method accomplished more than I first set out to achieve, which was to be able to lose weight at any time without going hungry and without restricting the kinds of foods I

ONE BOWL

1

eat. As you'll discover, controlling body weight is only one aspect of my discovery. How does One Bowl eating do all this? I can tell you up front that it has nothing to do with counting or even thinking about calories. Nor does it have to do with becoming aware of the nutritional values of food. You're going to find that the One Bowl method challenges conventional wisdom in a variety of ways, for it places no controls whatsoever on the food available to you in the world. Having lived according to this system for over two decades now, I can eat any food that I really want. Yet I automatically eat in a nourishing way, one that is literally satisfying to body, soul, and psyche.

In order to accomplish these things, I pay close attention to the sensation of hunger in my body. This familiar sensation is the opening note of what soon becomes a whole symphony of inner sensations associated with my natural digestive processes. When I sit down to eat a meal, this symphony of inner sensations begins, and it continues as long as I'm eating. It is literally the background music of my body's life. Unfortunately, most of us are so busy talking, or thinking about something else during our meals, that we don't even hear the opening chord of this inner symphony. When we eat, our attention is drawn to the people or activities around us. Maybe we are disciplining the children, watching television, reading the morning paper, reading a book, listening to the stock market report, or playing computer games. In this increasingly fast-paced world, it is not unusual to eat at the office desk. A young woman who is employed as an advertising rep for a radio station in Phoenix recently boasted to me that she had learned to eat every kind of food in the world—including Chinese with chopsticks—while driving in her car locked in freeway traffic! Under these stressful conditions, it is impossible to listen to your body's needs.

You may be surprised when I say that if you are really into the culinary arts, you may be so deeply involved with the tastes, textures, and aromas of your food that you don't hear a single note of the subtle, inner symphony that can tell you so much about how your body is responding to the food you are shoving into your face.

No wonder so many people in our society are suffering from food-related diseases, ranging from chronic indigestion to obesity and clogged arteries! We eat for convenience and we eat for comfort but we don't pay attention to ourselves while we do it. According to a *USA Today* report, published on October 27, 1999, the number of Americans considered obese (more than 30% over their ideal body weight) has skyrocketed from one in eight to one in five! The next time you go to the mall or to church, look around you at all those big waistlines. Even in this age of the workout, the

ONE BOWL

American people are becoming increasingly overweight. I submit that the most important consideration about obesity is not an aesthetic one, however, but a symptom that we are totally out of touch with our relationship to food.

Breaking old habits, especially well-established eating habits, is not easy. But I am proposing that there is a way to eat that lets you rediscover a natural and harmonious relationship to eating—just by becoming aware of certain internal sensations, sensations which you may not be aware of. Whether you come to this book for help controlling your body weight or for discovering the broader benefits of greater food awareness, the benefits the One Bowl system offers are nothing less than a vastly improved lifestyle.

It sounds simple enough as an idea—and once you become adept at it, nothing could be simpler. But the One Bowl method will demand a few things from you: a little discipline, some new knowledge, some patience, and the time you need to find your way to the utter simplicity of this path.

I have discovered that when I pay attention to the symphony of my internal sensations, I learn that these signals from my body are telling me something important about the food I am eating. Like background music, these signals hover at the edge of my consciousness whenever I sit down to eat. They comprise a language that, once I learn to read it, is clear, accurate, and reliable.

I have discovered that I can listen to this inner music, learn to interpret its language, and literally be tutored by my own body on how to lose weight!

I have discovered that I can listen to this inner music, learn to interpret its language, and literally be tutored by my own body on what to eat so that I feel good all the time! Once I've achieved what my body (not my head) tells me is my ideal food intake, I can happily maintain that state of health, contentment, high level of functioning—and yes, my optimum weight—simply by continuing to listen to the same inner music each time I eat.

And of course, if I go through a busy or stressful period, during which time I am unable to attend to my inner signals, then I might gain a little weight, which is my signal that I am getting out of touch with what my body is telling me. But as soon as the stress is off, I return to the One Bowl method and I return to that level of awareness that allows me to choose exactly what and how I should eat. The extra pounds melting away are again my measure that I am back on my path.

When I started listening to my inner food symphony, one of the first principles I discovered was this:

> *I gain weight because my head*
> *makes food decisions that*
> *ignore what my body wants.*

I gain weight because my head makes food decisions that ignore what my body wants. As you read these words, keep in mind that this is about much more than how you look or how you fit in your clothes or how your measurements conform to the current social standards of beauty. Your weight is your barometer that tells you to pay attention to signals that your body is sending you about what it needs. You may not believe that your body can know what it needs, or that it can communicate its needs to you in a meaningful way. But it can and it does—continually. As you start exploring the One Bowl method, you will begin discovering things about your body and its natural relationship to food and to eating that you didn't know—things that are simple, profound, and effective.

If you are like most people, you probably have tried to follow various food systems, whether it was to manage a health problem, improve your energy levels, to honor a value system that was important to you, or even to gain weight because you were too thin. If you have read a few books on nutrition or dieting, you will have noticed that they all set their standards according to the needs of an idealized body, or of an "average" body (whatever that is), instead of teaching you how to pay attention to the deepest inner needs of your unique body. It's important to understand that the food scientists who do the research for most of these books usually build all their findings around what is a theoretical, idealized, or average body. In most cases, they use what in this age of computers we would call a "virtual body;" they define a theoretical body, a model that exists only in the computer as a set of laboratory theories based on scientific observation. You might even call it a computer-generated stereotype.

What's wrong with that? It is, after all, the basis of modern medicine. Nothing is wrong with it if your goal is to feed virtual bodies or computer-generated stereotypes. But if you are not one of these, how well will these programs work for you? What about your real body? Your very personal body? Your absolutely unique and individual body? The one you live in? What does it want?

The food recommendations for the average body that emerge from this virtual system amount to arbitrary restrictions that will ultimately leave you feeling unsatisfied, and even deprived of food. You may even feel that you are being punished when you try to follow the food plans prescribed. And what does anyone generally do when they feel unsatisfied, deprived, or persecuted? If you don't know the answer to that, rest assured that the fast food processors and marketers do. The answer? You reach for "comfort foods," the foods high in fats, sugar, and good old white flour. While these may satisfy a transient emotional need, the impact they have over time is likely to add to your feelings of dissatisfaction and disharmony.

Dietary systems based on virtual models of the human body all too often lead us to hopeless conflicts. We find ourselves having to choose between the foods we want to eat but can't allow ourselves to have without feeling guilty; or we eat what we want but watch our bodies grow larger and larger. Remember, weight gain is your barometer that something is amiss and it is a flag telling you, "Pay attention!" With the One Bowl method you will learn how to make contact with the digestive sensations and feelings continually occurring within your unique body. You will learn to hear this inner symphony, and then to understand what this music means to you in terms of your daily eating habits, your feelings about life, and your overall health.

*Once you begin eating by the
One Bowl method, you will notice
changes within three or four days.*

Once you begin eating by the One Bowl method, you will start noticing changes within three or four days. If you are overweight or underweight you will notice your body starting to move toward its optimal weight within ten days. When I first started this plan, twenty-plus years ago, I was amazed at the changes that I was experiencing. Remember, I started it to lose weight, and I did—in fact, I lost twenty pounds in about ten weeks. But that was only the beginning, for I was feeling better, had more energy, and felt a sense of harmony, balance, and personal satisfaction that I hadn't experienced in years.

As you embark on this method it is important to remember that any concern with weight—whether you are trying to lose it or gain it—should be perceived in a very different way than you may have perceived it in the past. It is your barometer of how much or how little you are in touch with your body's own signals to you. In the One Bowl method your natural weight range is not a numerical goal to be achieved by something you do. It is not a fixed number on an insurance report, or a column on an HMO's chart. One Bowl

ONE BOWL

asks that you give up all your previous notions about your ideal body weight being a standard that some person or some institution, or even the latest fashion magazine, has established. Rather, the secret of your success with this method is the discovery of a body size and weight that is completely congruent with who you are—your personal constitution and your wholeness as a unique being. If you have some image or idea of a weight or size you'd like to be that is different from this congruency—perhaps smaller— you may very well end up working against the natural processes of your personal evolution to try to achieve those results. The body does not want to be denied and if you try to force it, there will be a price to pay later on. By contrast, One Bowl promotes congruence with your true self in the present moment, day by day.

People with chronic complaints associated with eating and digestion, such as burping, gas, bad teeth, heartburn, acid stomach, bad breath, stomachaches, and chronic constipation or diarrhea, can use this book to begin to understand their symptoms in a new way. People who regularly use enzyme supplements, or one of the many doctor-prescribed or over-the-counter antacids, may discover that the One Bowl method can end this dependency.

Two years ago I spoke with a man who had been spending nearly $150 a month on medical checkups and prescriptions for antacids and laxatives. After trying the One Bowl method for six

ONE BOWL

weeks he started cutting back on the prescriptions and eventually he stopped their use entirely. After a consultation with his physician, the two of them working together figured out that this man's habit of eating a diet of highly processed foods when he was stressed, together with taking the prescribed antacids and laxatives, were in fact causing his problems! Today he is comfortable with his lifestyle, his body and his diet, and he is $150 per month richer because he no longer has to buy antacids and laxatives. And, oh yes, he is also twenty pounds lighter!

The One Bowl method demonstrates a truth as old as Creation itself—but largely unknown to modern medicine—that the body, your body, knows what it needs to be healthy, and that the many sensations, discomforts and symptoms you experience are not signs of disease so much as signals from your body reporting on its internal state.

The One Bowl method demonstrates a truth as old as Creation itself—but largely unknown to modern medicine—that the body, your body, knows what it needs to be healthy, and that the many sensations, discomforts, and symptoms you experience are not signs of disease so much as signals from your body reporting on its internal state. If you experience signals of distress, it is for a good reason and the worst thing you can do is block them with drugs. If you follow the One Bowl method for learning to listen to and heed your inner signals, you will learn how to make better decisions about your general health.

If my claims sound too wonderful, miraculous, or ridiculous to you, rest assured that you are mirroring the fact that you don't believe in or trust the healing abilities and decision-making powers inherent in the human body—in your own body! I do not mean this in a negative or reproachful way at all. Our entire culture actively discourages any of us from gaining true knowledge about our bodies and instead leads us to distrust ourselves. Sadly, the medical profession, and particularly those associated with the food industry, are some of the worst offenders.

Nowhere are we taught that our bodies can regulate or heal themselves. Yet they do. As one enlightened physician once told me, "Life on this planet would have been impossible without the capacity of our bodies to self-heal and self-regulate." Consider how your body maintains a perfect heart rate, a certain temperature range, how it extracts micro-nutrients and sends them flowing into the blood stream to carry the fuel for mobilizing our cells. The human organism silently maintains an enormous symphony of operations which keep the healthy body in homeostasis (functioning within a normal and healthy range). When the stresses of living cause it to begin to get out of balance in some way, signals of distress appear. The wise person listens to those signals and simply makes the necessary corrections. One Bowl can start you on that healing path.

If our bodies are designed, as I say, to communicate information to us about what we need, why don't we just naturally and automatically listen to them? Why don't we heed these messages? Part of the answer to these questions can be found in the rigors and demands of society itself. As little children sitting in classrooms, we were repeatedly told to "control" ourselves. "Sit up straight!" "Pay attention" (which meant pay attention to the teacher or other adults). And "behave" (which meant to act according to standards established by someone else, usually an adult).

Continuing with these childhood rules, we spend our young lives trying to meet the strict standards and expectations of our families, our schools, our bosses, and our government, so that eventually we set up within ourselves impossible and deadly standards of behavior that may have very little to do with what our bodies actually need. And the further we get from our bodies' own inner signals, the more we tend to force ourselves to make special adjustments to meet inhuman and unhealthy social and economic goals imposed from outside us.

Unfortunately, the human organism just doesn't follow external social standards or arbitrary rules established for one person's convenience or economic gain. It just does not work that way, and trying to force your body to meet standards that cause it to be stressed leads to conflict, frustration, and then disease. The human organism has its own rhythms and standards to follow; these are based on maintaining the health of each and every cell that is a part of the whole. The human organism is flexible and miraculously adaptable, but it has its limits. If those limits are not respected because you are not listening to the signals, then the organism begins to break down. First this might manifest only in subtle ways, such as increased fatigue, or by gaining or losing weight, or through indigestion, or chronic tension. If you are the person living in such a body and you continue to ignore these signals of distress, the signals will escalate into symptoms, manifesting as everything from indigestion to cancer, heart disease, and eventually to an early death.

I am convinced that if we habitually try to control nature instead of listening to it and cooperating with it, and if we ignore our healthy limits and push beyond them with pills and various regimens for diet, exercise, work, or even play, we will be rewarded with a short, frustrating, and uncomfortable life.

How many of us were taught early in our lives that our inner feelings and sensations were the signals by which our organism's regulation and healing is effected? In modern life in the Western World, the answer to that is "almost no one." On the contrary, we were taught to ignore our inner signals in favor of obeying various "outer authorities," experts, and specialists. But what can they really know about the uniqueness that is you or me?

If you are to understand the One Bowl method and begin applying it in your life, you will have to face these issues head on. It would be irresponsible of me not to mention that developing a trust for your inner feelings will sometimes put you in the position of having to challenge some authority, or work against some pretty powerful forces in our culture. Ultimately you may have to choose between the certainty of your own inner sensations and the arbitrary authority of cultural conventions established by someone else's life experience or research.

The One Bowl method invites you to live this bold statement:

> You are the primary source;
> your body is the living experience.
> Trust it, go with it.

Each of us experiences life on three levels simultaneously: at a cortical level (I think and reflect); at a hormonal level (I feel and experience); at a molecular level (I pulsate and move). However, our language does not allow us to say *I am* in a way that we know, beyond a shadow of a doubt, that we are talking about all three of these levels simultaneously. And yet, we are all of those levels, functioning in unison every single moment we live. And because we have no way to simply express this vital unison, we tend to think of ourselves in fragments or divisions. We say *my this* or *my that,* but must qualify what we are saying by adding *my body* or *my feelings,* as if these parts of ourselves were somehow different and apart, not joined as the coherent and continuous whole that is really us.

You may find this a lot to think about, especially in terms of making decisions about how you eat. But looking at how we think about ourselves provides important clues about what's wrong, as well as guidelines for effecting change. The simple truth is, our very language perpetuates an artificial split between our bodies and our minds. This split makes it difficult to trust the kinds of inner signals that I have been describing. As you read on, I would like you to keep in mind that when I say *me, my body, you, your body,* I am always referring to the whole person, the physical, emotional, mental, and spiritual organism that is you or me in all of our glorious wholeness.

By now you may be asking, *Is all this philosophy necessary?* And I would answer you—yes it is! The One Bowl eating method is simplicity itself but in order to adopt it you will have to stop and think about what you are eating, and how you eat it. If that is philosophy, then so be it.

There are certainly plenty of ways to become more conscious of the meaning of food in our lives without giving so much effort to thinking about it. If you have stomach distress or are otherwise uncomfortable with your body, just pop a pill, right? But if you are reading this book I suspect that you already know that such methods don't work, at least not for long. By pursuing the One Bowl method and the philosophy that supports it, you will discover important relationships between how, when, and what you eat, and achieving greater comfort throughout your entire life. One Bowl promotes a different way of making choices. It invites you to discard the external voice of authority and live from the *inner authority* of your own body and soul.

The One Bowl method can be a way out of many types of food problems, some of which you may be experiencing. If you follow me in the One Bowl journey, along the way you will gain a new trust in the power and wisdom that you possess within your own body.

Food is both my daily sustenance and a group of ideas that are intimately connected with my way of being in the world. Food defines the boundaries of my personality, expressing who I am, what I want in life, and even how I go about trying to get what I want. And since eating is one way I make my being grow, I cannot eat without experiencing many strong feelings, consciously or unconsciously, about myself, about what I am eating, and about the environment and conditions under which I eat. Let me say that again:

> Since eating is one way I make my being grow, I cannot eat without experiencing many strong feelings, consciously or unconsciously, about myself, about what I am eating, and about the environment and conditions under which I eat.

When and how often I feel hungry, what I choose to eat, and how my body uses food—all of these are expressions of my individual self.

If it is true that I eat because I am hungry, but also to affirm my being, my personality, my sense of life, it should be no surprise that eating would also be an important emotional experience. Each bite of food that I take initiates dozens of tiny reactions in every part of my being, including and especially concentrating on my digestive system. From my lips to my intestines I experience fluid secretions, sensations of motion and weight, changes in energy, feelings of pleasure, and just below my conscious perceptions, chemical adjustments and increased molecular activity. These changes seem to me as complex as a symphony, with many individual parts of my organism working together to make the music harmonious.

This same food symphony goes on within you of course, though you may have been too busy to notice it. The One Bowl method begins by insulating you from external noise so that you can pay attention to your internal food symphony; then it shows you how to interpret and evaluate these sounds for the important signals they are.

I used to eat mostly with my head, paying attention primarily to the ideas running through my mind while I was eating. If I was eating with another person, I paid more attention to whatever we were talking about than I did to the food I was eating. Sometimes I was focused on the taste of my food, particularly if it was unusual or especially delicious, but I ignored that food entirely once I'd swallowed it. I almost always ate with other people, and I felt deprived or even embarrassed when I had to eat alone. I frequently combined eating and business. In fact, in the years that I was a publisher, the proverbial "publisher's lunch" was much more the rule than the exception for me. And many times I followed the publisher's lunch with a publisher's dinner that same day, entertaining my authors and friends in style. I was at the height of my professional life.

But that wasn't all. Though I didn't realize it at the time, I was also completely out of touch with my own inner processes. My weight was only a symptom of that, the barometer that I refused to heed. I had no idea that there was such a thing as inner processes, that is, an inner reality that makes me who I am. Only after I began using the One Bowl method did I began to realize that those inner processes I was learning to experience actually were me!

The One Bowl method begins
by isolating you from external noise
so that you can concentrate
on your internal symphony.

During this period in my life, my wife and I hired Robert, a natural foods gourmet chef, as our personal cook. Robert specialized in healthy and delicious vegetarian meals, meals that were carefully worked out according to principles of good nutrition which were hundreds of years old. Robert planned all of our menus, and at every meal he explained the menu to us. "This is the really healthy way to eat," he declared.

When I sat down to eat his food, I tried to recall what Robert had told me about the health values of the food he had prepared. And I did enjoy the flavors and textures of each meal. Robert was an excellent cook, no doubt about it! However, my whole relationship with the food he served me occurred from the neck up. It was all very healthy sounding, and nearly always a delicious eating experience. So, what was wrong, you say? I was paying little or no attention to what was going on below my neck—where my body accepted and digested the food I ate and assimilated it into my being.

As I would eventually learn when I started paying more attention to the food symphony in my body, my relationship to food and eating was in reality complex and ever-changing, and I became fascinated by this process. Eating was like carrying on an inner dialogue with myself at meals. I began to prefer to eat alone so that I could pay more attention to the food messages I was receiving about myself. And I no longer wanted to eat what other people, even a gourmet chef, might decide I should eat. I wanted to choose my own food—always.

There were times when the choices I made, and the needs I sought to satisfy through food, were purely emotional. At such times I might eat foods from my childhood or early adolescence. Having grown up in a small town in Texas, I might choose Tex-Mex at one meal and find that while I ate, memories from my early life, both the good and the bad, became aroused. At other times I would eat something that was totally healthy and wholesome, and come away from the experience feeling deeply satisfied at a molecular level. But whatever my choices, I always came away with new insights about my relationship to food and to eating.

While mine might be an unusual example, people who have adopted the One Bowl method have often said that, although the circumstances might be different for them, the core of their experience was quite similar to mine. Prior to trying the One Bowl method, they had focused their awareness on what they thought about the healthy value of food rather than on the actual experience of eating.

One woman, Barbara, recounted that in her workday world in real estate sales, she often had lunch, and sometimes even breakfast and dinner, with clients, co-workers, or other associates.

Although very successful in her work, she had grown extremely unhappy with how she felt and looked, and she admitted that she was feeling burned out. No wonder, since she was constantly feeling intestinal distress, was nearly forty pounds overweight, and had virtually no personal life outside of her work! Her doctor told her nothing was wrong with her that losing a few pounds wouldn't cure, and while her weight had flown out of control she also knew there was a lot more than that involved.

Barbara said that a friend gave her a copy of *One Bowl*. Soon after reading the book, which she admitted doing while she was eating her lunch, she realized that she never tasted her food or paid any attention to how she felt after eating. No wonder, since nearly every meal was dominated by either talking about real estate, thinking about the next sale, or eating at her desk while she did her paper work.

By its nature, selling real estate is a social business, with the added burden of extensive paper work, so at first Barbara didn't think it would be possible to eat alone or shift her mealtime activities so that she could stay more focused on her inner processes. But then she decided that for a few weeks she would not have any more dinner meetings. Instead, she began eating her evening meal by herself, following the One Bowl method. For this one meal a day, she ate alone and paid attention to eating. This soon became

ONE BOWL

2 3

a way for her to get in touch not only with her food but with herself—her inner processes—beginning with the taste but proceeding to chewing and swallowing, and going all the way to digestion. This led her to focus on her personal needs, which she realized for the first time that she had been neglecting.

The last time we talked, Barbara reported that she had lost ten or twelve pounds, and she was very happy about that. But she said that it was only a small portion of the benefits she had gained from following the One Bowl method. She was much more aware of the foods she really loved to eat now, not just because of their taste but because of how her body felt an hour, or even twenty-four hours, later. She was beginning to hear the inner symphony and was enjoying the music of her own life.

Barbara's story helped to confirm my own experiences, as well as the experiences of others who have followed the One Bowl method. Thanks to this way of eating, I am much more likely to eat with my whole body. I focus my attention on how well my body assimilates the food it receives. I choose foods it digests well. I now call eating with other people—social eating— "eating with my head" since my attention at such meals is always focused outside myself, on other people, or on their ideas. When I do social eating, I don't know what my body feels about the food I bring it. Often this leaves me with feelings of dissatisfaction later on, which

I pay careful attention to even hours later, because out of it often come insights about what transpired during that period of social eating.

I must confess however, that "whole body eating" takes more time than head eating does, particularly if you have been a person who is always eating on the run. Whole body eating—One Bowl eating—begins when you first feel hungry and ends only when digestion is complete. It includes becoming more aware of the demands of social eating and how it affects every aspect of food— from shared social interactions to the choices you make in the food you eat, how you hold your body while you eat, and how you feel two or three hours later. Through the many simple exercises found in this book you will be able to explore these ideas in greater detail.

SOCIAL EATING

EXERCISE:

> The purpose of this first exercise is to consciously and deliberately experience the distractions that normally take you away from paying attention to the experience of eating. You will exaggerate those distractions so that you can see them more clearly. This is a good place to

begin exploring the One Bowl method, since it highlights some of the problems with eating in your normal way—assuming your normal way is in a social situation. It is through our experiences that we can become more aware of ourselves, what we like, and what we'd like to change about the way we live.

The best way to do this exercise is while you are eating with friends, at a house not your own, or in a restaurant. Choose the same food as the other people eat, whether you want that food or not. If you are a vegetarian, eat chicken, fish or even red meat. If you ordinarily eat a typical American diet—such as meat and potatoes—try eating only vegetables. Or choose a food that you are not accustomed to eating or which you would never, in a million years, decide to eat otherwise. If you have a friend, or a partner who wants to do this experiment with you, go to a restaurant and each of you order something that you especially like but which you know the other person never orders. Then, when the food comes, trade plates.

Eat rapidly, and talk as fast as you can while eating. If you are eating in a restaurant and you have any say in the matter, choose a sports bar or micro-brewery since that type of restaurant is usually pretty noisy. Go there right at peak time, the lunch or dinner hour when the place will be jammed with people. Or go there during a major sports event when people are drinking, and are loud and boisterous. You can even ask someone in your party or the server for their food recommendations and order what they suggest instead of something you would ordinarily choose on your own. Or just arbitrarily decide to order whatever the person sitting across from you orders. When the meal is over and you have left the restaurant, take a moment to sit alone, then ask yourself how you feel.

To carry out this experiment at home, let someone else choose and prepare the food you will eat. Turn on both the TV and a radio. Crank up the volume, talk continuously while eating, or focus on something serious, such as the family finances, while you are eating. When the meal is over ask yourself how you liked what you experienced and how you feel now.

Did you receive any messages from your body regarding this experience of exaggerated social eating? If so, what are you feeling and where in your body are these feelings located? Maybe your stomach feels tight, or you still feel hungry even though you've just had a big meal. Maybe there's a sensation that you can't quite identify right away. Write all this information down on a piece of paper under the dated heading Social Eating. When you have answered these questions satisfactorily, and feel ready to move on, ask yourself, "Is this experience so different from the way I normally eat my meals?"

CHOICES AND INNER HARMONY

The more you make food choices that you genuinely like, and that your body likes, the more harmoniously and completely your body can make use of that food, leaving less of it to be stored as fat. This is a bold unscientific statement I admit, but it feels true to me and has proven to be the case with people who have followed the One Bowl method. One nutritional researcher pointed out that what could be operating here is the fact that stress factors can cause our bodies to store calories in greater abundance. Eating under stressful conditions, therefore—even stressful conditions which we enjoy—such as in a noisy, busy restaurant with friends, changes our biochemistry and alters how we digest and store our food.

However, it is your own unique experience that you will be interested in now. Focusing on the "science" of eating is actually

ONE BOWL

beside the point. The One Bowl method is aimed at learning more about what your body actually wants to eat at every meal.

The more you can become aware of the signals of hunger, and of the cessation of hunger, the less you will tend to overeat and the better your body will be able to process and make use of whatever you do eat.

The more you can become aware of the signals of hunger, and of the cessation of hunger, the less you will tend to overeat and the better your body will be able to process and make use of whatever you do eat. At first, when you try to pay attention to your internal signals, you may not know what it is you are looking for. But once you begin to recognize these simple sensations, you will find these signals easy to follow.

I should tell you that I am deliberately choosing *not* to give you too many hints about what you might experience when you do these exercises. The reason for this is that I don't want to give you ideas. Instead, I want to lead you to find your own experience. Your sensations are your sensations, and my suggestions about what you should or should not be experiencing might be more

ONE BOWL

2 9

misleading than helpful. Therefore I ask you to find your own way, working from the deliberately scanty clues I am providing.

As you begin the One Bowl method, you will discover that you experience more pleasure when you follow your internal signals than when you don't. Over a period of time, you will see that different foods, eaten at different times of the day, produce different effects on your body. These effects will vary according to the mood you're in and your body's physical needs. You will discover that eating has the power to change your mood. When you strive to eat foods that are compatible with your body's inner signals, the best internal music is made. Your body makes efficient use of your food no matter what it happens to be—whether fast food or healthy gourmet—and when that kind of harmony is achieved, your mood will either remain good or get better.

As I was writing this, the word "congruence" came to mind. My dictionary defines congruence as the quality or state of being in harmony or agreement. When you follow the One Bowl method, you will gradually experience more congruence between your body and the choices you make concerning how and what you eat. You will find yourself changing your habits so that the food you eat will be more harmonious with your inner processes. You will modify your present diet, but you'll do it gently, at your own pace and in accordance with your own inner signals, not because of someone's analysis, instructions, model, or research.

The changes you will make can be as gradual as you wish. Since they are dependent on the unique signals you receive from within yourself, and on your interpretation of them, you will always be in complete control.

Once you realize that this method really gives you more control over your life, from the issue of body weight, to the "pep" or energy you have, to your mood and general outlook on life—all through the food you eat—your sense of contentment, personal power, and wellbeing will rise. You will be able to stabilize your body weight so that it is congruent with who you are, while pleasing all your other (emotional) requirements about food. In this respect, One Bowl is about food attitudes; it demonstrates that as your attitudes toward food change, so will your relationship to your body and to the world around you.

> *One Bowl is about food attitudes;*
> *it demonstrates that, as your*
> *attitudes toward food change,*
> *so will your relationship to your body*
> *and the world around you.*

ONE BOWL

In the social eating exercise, I recommended that you write down what you experienced when you ate food deliberately selected by someone else in a noisy place. This act of recording your experiences with the One Bowl method can be a real eye-opener. If you feel comfortable using a journal to record your thoughts and feelings, now is a good time to locate a little book that will become your Food Awareness Journal. Be sure to take your time looking for a special book that you will use. It will contain your most intimate food thoughts. Exploring and recording this vital information is a sacred process, and it demands a wonderful journal to record these things in.

Because you will be recording experiences about your thoughts, feelings, and insights as you go along, make sure that the book invites you to write in it. Don't choose a journal that would please someone else—just please yourself. These will be your thoughts, your feelings, your experiences and yours only and everything about the book you write in should encourage that.

There are many beautiful journals available in bookstores and stationery stores these days, so take your time locating one that

ONE BOWL

you'll be happy with. Find one that pleases you to pick up, hold, look at, touch, and write in.

After you have found the journal that's just right, make it your own. Add decorations to it inside or out; color it, paint it, title it, draw in it, record other very important items in it, scribble in it, do whatever feels right and will help to make that journal absolutely, uniquely yours.

As you set out to record your food discoveries, decide on how you are going to do that. For example, some people choose to keep their notes in order by exercise or by date while others might divide the book up into separate sections, allotting so many pages for each. And some people make their entries totally at random. If you keep sections, you might, for example, have one for food lists. Within that section you might compile a list of foods at the outset that you know nearly always bring you a sense of inner harmony; another list might include foods you find delicious but which ultimately leave you feeling inharmonious. You might also make lists for foods that really touch off bad feelings in you physically or emotionally, and a list of foods that you know you are allergic to. In this way, using whatever lists or other means occur to you, you will begin to construct a map of your upcoming food exploration journeys.

One person, Amy, who is also a poet, likes to write little vignettes in her journal about preparing and eating meals that are particularly memorable for her. These vignettes always include her reflections on the total eating experience, from food preparation, which she loves to do, through insights associated with the food she makes and the feelings she has during and after eating. Amy is a person who enjoys her solitude and whose poetry is deeply personal and yet lyrical. Being private and somewhat protective about her food journal, she didn't want to share her writings with us in these pages, but she did say it was fine to share this idea for making journal entries.

As you read through this book, think about the areas of eating that are most important to you. Record your experiences with the exercises any way that feels right: by date, in random order, by subject, or by following the outline of this book. Trust what your inner self seems to want. Remember, no one has ever gone where you are about to go. Your upcoming food awareness explorations will be absolutely unique. They are yours alone to enjoy. Your Food Awareness Journal can become a big part of your One Bowl process. Cherish and honor it.

CHOOSE A BOWL

Okay. We have the preliminaries out of the way and now you are ready to make food awareness explorations a part of your everyday life. What is the first thing to do? The first changes you will make are not in the foods you eat. Instead, you will be focusing on your eating patterns—that set of habits you have developed over the years which determines *how rather than what you eat*. Through this shift in focus you will begin to see the food you eat in a new way. Putting the spotlight on *how* rather than *what* you eat is a key part of the One Bowl method. Consider it as a food adventure that you will be taking with me.

You'll begin this adventure by choosing a single bowl from which to eat. One of the early enthusiasts of the One Bowl method was a woman who led people on treks into wilderness areas in the Rocky Mountains. She said that when she was advising her clients on the best equipment to bring on a backpacking trip, she told each of them to bring along a single metal cup from which to eat. Obviously, she wanted them to have a metal bowl because it wouldn't break. She told them that part of their adventure would be to look upon themselves as going on a kind of spiritual mission, or a mission of self-discovery. This would require them to leave behind old habits in favor of discovering new things about themselves and their relationship to nature. She liked to use the example of Siddhartha, the founder of Buddhism, who left behind his life as the son of a nobleman, equipped himself with little more than a single bowl and the clothes on his back, and ventured forth into the world to seek deeper understanding.

While we may not all be like Siddhartha, setting out on lofty spiritual missions, there is a common thread of self-discovery in my friend's advice to her clients as they set off into the wilderness. As you set off on your One Bowl food exploration, I want you to choose a single bowl from which to eat. This means temporarily giving up eating from a plate in your normal manner. Instead, you will eat your meals only from the bowl you've chosen for this quest. You will use your bowl extensively during this initial learning period, to help you learn to keep your attention focused on your internal food messages.

Eating from your bowl in this way will both enclose and personalize your food experience. One person told me that by always eating from a single bowl, she found a way of "containing," her eating experience. She chose a bowl made by a local potter whose work she really liked. "It delights me just to hold it in my hand," she said. "And when I eat from it, I am reminded of the special meanings— that how we eat and what we eat are unique to each of us."

I like this example because it emphasizes how the bowl helps us focus on the highly personal nature of the foods we enjoy and choose to incorporate into our beings.

Once you have chosen a bowl you like, try to stick with it. Use the same bowl whenever you eat by the One Bowl method. In time the use of this bowl will take on its own special meaning for you.

ONE BOWL

So the first part of this exercise—finding a bowl that works for you, that will allow you to bring a highly personal framework to the experience of eating—is definitely important.

But before you set out in search of the perfect bowl, take this idea one step further. Look for a bowl that you can comfortably hold in your hand. Yes, that's right. Use a bowl you can hold in your hand while you eat. The reason for this is that if you have a bowl that will sit on the table, then you can also leave it on the table. If you can leave it on the table, then you are more likely to fall back into your old habit of focusing on something or someone else in your environment besides the food you are eating and the sensations of digestion occurring inside you.

The act of holding your bowl as you eat is important since it involves your whole body in the process, requiring you to focus your attention not just on getting the forkful of food from the bowl to your mouth but also on coordinating bowl and fork. One man pointed out to me that eating in this way—with the bowl in one hand and the eating utensil in the other—is suggestive of the whole process of giving and receiving that was an important lesson in his own eating experience.

Ideally, you should find a special bowl, one that does not have a base on it, but that has a rounded bottom instead. This special bowl should please you by its appearance so that you will feel happy eating from it, and it should feel good to hold in your hand. If you cannot find such a bowl right away, make a point of eating from whatever bowl you have as if it required you to hold it, that is, remembering the giving and receiving cycle suggested by eating in this way.

The bowl that I began this work with was rather small—about three and one-half inches across at the mouth, and with a heavy, rounded bottom. Your bowl should be large enough to comfortably hold at least one cup of food, but not more than a cup and a half. The way to tell if the size is right is easy—just pour a measuring cup's worth of water into it and see how much it will hold.

If you can find a suitable bowl around the house, use it. If not, definitely go out and search for something wonderful. And remember, it is important to treat yourself. Find a bowl you will really like—a bowl that seems just right for you. When you go shopping for this bowl, look at antique bowls, bowls from romantic places, contemporary ceramic bowls, clear glass bowls and even children's bowls (which can be delightfully playful). Over the years I have accumulated a small collection—one of each.

If you do not have a round-bottomed bowl, but you have internet capability, visit my One Bowl website. And by the way, if you mistakenly type in www.onebowl.com, you will get Kraft Foods—

which you will quickly recognize is not me. My One Bowl internet address is www.onebowlbook.com.

At my One Bowl website I feature the beautiful and unique, handmade, round-bottomed bowls of artist Anne Franklin. Anne has created a line of ceramic, round-bottomed bowls especially for use with the One Bowl method. These bowls each hold about one and a half cups of food, just the right amount. In addition, they are powerful spiritual objects in their own right, and they feel great in your hand. Anne's bowls are moderately priced; no two of them are exactly alike.

If you use a bowl with a standard base, use it as if it had no base. This means holding it in your hand while you eat and never setting it down on the table! If you leave the table during your meal for any reason, such as to answer the phone, carry your bowl with you! The point is to maintain your link with your food and with the One Bowl method of eating by preserving your connection with the bowl continuously during your meal.

It may be easy to forget this because, in the American culture, everyone eats from a plate set on the table in front of them. This style of eating is deeply ingrained in us all. If you continue the practice of eating from a plate on the table, you will be reinforcing your old eating habits, and nullifying the One Bowl method even

though you practice all the other parts of it. So, if you possibly can, make your break from the plate.

Even though you may be excited to get started using this method, it is important not to hurry the bowl-choosing process. Remember, you are seeking the *right* bowl, that one perfect bowl from which you will eat each day. You are seeking the bowl that calls to you, the bowl that sings to you, the bowl that is you. This is a sacred container. It will be your primary tool for transforming your food life.

Just as you are a unique individual in the world, so your bowl should mirror your uniqueness. One Bowl does not begin when you start eating; it begins when you decide to search for a bowl that is just right for you. Choosing the right bowl is an aesthetic decision that will involve your whole being just as eating will begin to involve your whole being. When you think you have found the right bowl, ask your stomach whether it likes what you have chosen, and write down your stomach's answer in your Food Awareness Journal! After all, you do not want to make such an important decision as choosing your bowl with your head alone.

Eating is a process of possession,
of receiving something from
the outside world and
incorporating it into yourself.

EATING IS A PROCESS OF POSSESSION

If you think about it, eating is a process of possession, of receiving something from the outside world and incorporating it into yourself, of taking that which is not you and receiving it within your boundaries. Your bowl becomes the first step in this process. Placing the food into your bowl announces to the world that it is now in your possession, to be received into your body for the purpose of nourishing you, pleasuring you, and providing you with the energy to do whatever it is you do in the world. Each time you put food into your bowl, you are making it your possession and preparing it for a vital inner transformation that will sustain your life.

Every culture has rituals that acknowledge the significance of this event, including elaborate and careful washing of face and hands before eating (the Middle East), tradition-bound forms for food preparation and presentation (the Orient), and the ritual of the place setting and the act of saying grace (European and American).

In modern life, the packaging of food and the commercial emphasis on food as entertainment is a kind of ritual, but it has taken us further and further from our primal sources, that is, the plants and animals which actually nourish us. Young people in America and Europe today, for the first time in human history, have no physical contact with the plants and animals that sustain their lives. They need never see or handle living animals but just buy them ready to eat from the fast food vendors. The continuing evolution of food technology means that young people are cut off from the source of their own sustenance.

Hal Zina Bennett tells in one of his books how early cultures who lived in harmony with the land held the sources of their food to be sacred. When harvesting vegetables, they performed elaborate rituals of thanks to the Earth, some of which lasted for days. When a hunter killed a wild animal for food, he and those who ate it gave thanks to the spirit of that animal for its sacrifice, even acknowledging it as a being like themselves. In most cases, these cultures based their dances and their sacred icons on the hunting and gathering of food, which were the core activities in their societies. But how do most Americans hunt and gather their food today? Write your thoughts about this in your Food Awareness Journal. Think about how the process of gathering and hunting comes up in your life, and what feelings you have in regard to those activities.

While I don't advocate that you return to primitive agrarian practices, the knowledge of these ancient customs will help remind you that eating involves your whole being. Eating is not simply a way to fill a void, or a way to make your stomach stop growling. It is a sacred act, one that is shared by all living beings on our planet. In a sense, you could say that everyone's lives derive from one bowl.

The physical bowl that you
have chosen to eat from
is a symbol for that greater
spiritual bowl which accompanies
the essence and meaning of your life.

The physical bowl that you have chosen to eat from is a symbol for that greater spiritual bowl which accompanies the essence and meaning of your life. Your bowl symbolizes your right to eat, your right to renew your life. You will find that eating in this way is deeply sustaining. The more frequently I eat from my bowl, the more I feel and enjoy the power of this simple truth.

HOLD THE BOWL IN YOUR HAND

While you eat, hold your bowl in one hand. If you normally eat with a utensil in your right hand, hold your bowl in

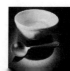

your left. If your bowl full of food feels too heavy to hold, rest your hand on the table or on your lap as you eat. It is permitted to rest your bowl while you chew and swallow, then raise the bowl to your mouth oriental-style each time you take a bite.

But before using your bowl for the first time, take a few minutes to get to know it. Grip it, pick it up, hold it in your eating hand. Your eating hand is the one which will hold the bowl of food; the hand you will eat with is your utensil hand. If you are left-handed you will probably use your right hand to hold the bowl.

So, before eating, hold your bowl, turn it over, examine it thoroughly. Test it in your hand. Admire its color, its texture, the weight of it. Do you like the glaze on it? Is it shiny or matte? Is it finished in your favorite color, or at least a color that pleases you? Record what you discover in your Food Awareness Journal.

A PRACTICE RUN

EXERCISE:

At some time when you are not preparing to eat, take a practice run with your new bowl. Go into your kitchen, into either the cabinets or the refrigerator, and find some food which you would like to eat. Put that food into your bowl. Now heft the bowl in your eating hand.

Full of food, how does your bowl look? Is it attractive, inviting? How does it feel? Are there any unusual associations you have with the bowl or the food in it? Write down whatever discoveries you make about your bowl in your Food Awareness Journal.

Once you have chosen a bowl, and feel ready to use it, begin in this way: Use the bowl at every meal just the way you have always used a plate. If for breakfast you usually eat bacon and eggs, put your bacon and eggs in your bowl and then eat them. Yes, and the toast, too. Put it right in there. If for lunch you eat a sandwich, put your sandwich into your bowl before you eat it. If for dinner you eat pork chops, mashed potatoes and gravy, and a vegetable, put them into your bowl.

Oops, hold it right there! Put a sandwich in my bowl? Certain foods do not fit easily into a bowl, and a sandwich is definitely one of them. Trying to get a sandwich to fit down into your bowl might make you feel foolish, irritated, or even disgusted. This ridiculous idea might even be enough to get you to stop using the One Bowl method altogether. Don't do that. Instead, stop reading. Take a deep breath. Calm yourself. Okay, that's better.

ONE BOWL

Let me explain. I have several good reasons for asking you to put everything you eat into your bowl, even your sandwiches. First, putting all the food you eat into your bowl will make the sacred act of eating more evident and visible to you. You will have to pay more attention to your food if it's all going to go into your bowl first.

Second, because a bowl does not allow you to keep different foods in your possession separate as they do on a plate, you will have to put less food into your bowl at any one time. Some foods, such as bacon and eggs, will combine just fine, while others—involving gravy or soup—will not. This means that you will not be able to place all the food you formerly put on a plate into your bowl at the same time. Instead, you will probably have to choose to keep your food more separate, maybe putting only one or two foods into your bowl at any one time.

You have no doubt noticed that your bowl is much smaller than most dinner plates are and will not hold even half as much food as you are used to eating. This means that you will be forced to have less food in your possession at any one time. It also means that, using your bowl, you will be less likely to overeat than you were when you "cleaned your plate." And you might also experience some anxiety surrounding the issue of food possession.

ONE BOWL

x

x

While the people you normally eat with are piling their plates high with food, you will be able to put only a much smaller portion of food into your bowl. Does this mean that you will not get enough to eat? For the moment, accept the fact that there will be less food in your bowl, and try to relax. Allow yourself to have second helpings and note the various feelings that may come up for you in the process of contemplating this change. Awareness of your anxiety around food—if you do happen to experience it—may turn out to be just as important as the other insights you might have in the days ahead. Write down any discoveries you have made concerning anxiety about not having enough food in your Food Awareness Journal. By the way, my solution to the problem of the sandwich being too large for your bowl is to cut the sandwich into pieces, then put the pieces into the bowl.

SITTING DOWN TO EAT

The seemingly simple act of sitting down with family or friends to eat, giving some sort of blessing for the meal, then taking a moment to observe all the food spread on the table before you, is an ancient and profound ritual. In the simplest sense it means, "I can survive." In a more profound sense it means, "I am blessed with this abundance." Take a moment to enjoy the special event of sharing a meal with others in this way. If any thoughts or feelings emerge, take note of them so that you can write them down in your Food Awareness Journal later.

I have often noticed that when people sit down to eat, they regard the food on the table before them as a gift, a portion of which they are certain to receive and possess. This is as it should be. One is used to surveying plates piled high with food, or seeing a table filled with plates of food, and immediately we get a sense that some or all of that food is our possession, that it is ours to enjoy.

At such moments, the look on most people's faces is definitely that of looking forward to partaking of this gift. It mirrors the expectation, the anticipation, of acquiring a new possession and incorporating it into our lives. This sense is strongest at special holidays, and most obvious on those holidays closely associated with food—in the Western culture these are birthdays, Christmas, Easter, Passover, and Thanksgiving. Can you get in touch with the special feelings of anticipation and fulfillment that are so prevalent on these days? I call these special moments *food events*. These food events are often filled with hidden or maybe not so hidden emotions. If they happen to coincide with your first explorations of the One Bowl method, food events are a good way to study the great variety of emotional associations you may have with food. Can you allow yourself to participate fully in food events? What do you receive besides the food itself when you take part in these events? Write your thoughts about this in your Journal.

Kirk was a man in his early thirties who contacted me regarding his insights during a family food event. Being Jewish, he had attended a seder, or Passover banquet, given by a new friend of his. While the food, the company, and the rituals were wonderful, reconnecting him with his cultural traditions and his history, he found himself feeling quite uncomfortable and even ambivalent about being there. To counteract some of his discomfort, he focused as much attention as he could on his eating experience, which he'd been learning to do with the help of One Bowl in the weeks prior to the event. But halfway through the seder he realized that his stomach was churning and he was feeling a combination of sadness, anger, and guilt.

Kirk sat through the whole event and managed to stay sociable and upbeat throughout. But when he got home, he wrote in his food journal until 3:00 A.M. Kirk re-experienced a complex of emotional associations with Passover banquets that he had attended as a child. While his mother was a religious Jew, his father took the position that all the old traditions were a bunch of nonsense and should be left in the past. Even so, Kirk's mother insisted on celebrating the holidays. Kirk's father usually made fun of them, though he participated by eating the food.

As he reflected on these past events, Kirk realized that he always overate at any food event he attended, Jewish or not, and that this same pattern of overeating had started with his family seders. He said that he felt torn in his loyalties at those times between his mother's commitment to upholding old traditions and his father's position that they were "old fashioned" and worthless. Kirk realized that elaborate food events were overlaid with such a complexity of thoughts, feelings, and sensations that he was hardly ever aware of the food he ate as anything other than something to quiet his anxiety and grief. The key sensation he associated with all food was a knot in his belly, and indigestion following any meal that involved more than two or three people.

For the next few days, Kirk noticed some carryover from these sensations and feelings even when he ate alone. Inspired by these insights, he knew that by following the One Bowl method he was on the right track. As he continued to pursue a greater understanding of his relationship to food, he eventually achieved a deeper calmness about eating and even lost the extra pounds that had motivated his quest in the first place.

EXERCISE:

Since our associations with food are often linked with family celebrations, especially around special holidays and family gatherings, remembering these often provides us with insights into eating patterns in our everyday lives. As in Kirk's example above, this area of experience can be a wellspring of information, telling us not only about our food choices but about mental, physical, and spiritual responses associated with eating.

Make a list in your Food Awareness Journal of the food events that are celebrated in your family. How are they different from the food events celebrated by your spouse's family, or a close friend's family? Your list might include Saturdays or Sundays, birthdays, Hanukkah, Passover, Easter, The Day of the Dead, Thanksgiving, Cinco de Mayo, and so forth. These are some of the more obvious food events; try to go beyond them to list food events that are unique to your life, your family heritage and any religious affiliations you might have.

Just record these notes in your Journal. It is not neces-

ONE BOWL

sary to analyze them or try to reason out why they are or are not significant in your present life. In fact, it's better if you don't try to analyze them in this way. The information you are putting together here is best handled intuitively, allowing your consciousness to put the pieces together for you without imposing interpretive methods that you may have learned from books, workshops, or classes you've taken. However, rest assured that the heightened awareness that you will achieve by writing down recollections of family food experiences will open new doors of awareness for you as you proceed with the One Bowl method.

THE WISDOM OF THE BOWL

Now that you have your bowl, what's going to happen to your sense of food possession—your personal daily food event—when all you have to eat is one small bowl of food? Especially if everyone else sitting at the table with you has a large plate of food? This can be a dilemma. Some people even consider it a serious problem. At first you might feel that you are going to be left out, that there is no way you can possess as much food as the rest of

ONE BOWL

the people at the table. One person described their first encounter with this situation as follows: "There I sat with my one little bowl in my hand, feeling like a beggar waiting for a handout!" By contrast, another person said, "As I held the bowl in my hand I felt it gave focus to the whole experience for me."

Expand and redirect your sense of food possession beyond your bowl.

If you feel more like the former than the latter person, expand and redirect your sense of food possession beyond your bowl. Instead of focusing on the your previous perception of possessing only what is on your plate, expand this sense of possession to cover the entire table of food before you. If you are eating with other people, and they are using plates, their sense of possession will be confined to their plates while yours can cover the entire table. You are not limited to the food that's presently in your bowl. This is a small perceptual shift but it's all-important. In the process, you have given yourself permission to range over all the free food—that is, food on the table which is not already on other people's plates. I will describe how I extend my sense of food possession to the entire table, and even beyond the table, in the section called Hunting.

ONE BOWL

EXERCISE:

The purpose of this exercise is to get in touch with how the sense of food possession has worked in your life. To do that, you will go back in memory to a special food event that you participated in.

Imagine for a minute that you are sitting at the table with the person or people with whom you normally share a meal—most likely your family, your spouse, or some friends. Just imagine the beginning of a typical meal at your house.

Food is piled into bowls and serving platters, filling the center of the table. Let's consider the dynamics that are at play in this scenario. The food is in the middle of the table and empty plates and utensils are set in front of every person, creating a place setting. The place settings also contain empty chairs. The empty chairs are carefully pushed right up to the table, one in front of each place setting. This setup is also part of the ritual of food possession.

Note what makes up a place setting: There is a knife, a fork, and a spoon, nearly always placed in a particular order. There may be other utensils to handle special foods. If meat is served, each person might receive a sharp cutting knife. In addition, there might be a small fork for appetizers, an extra fork for a salad, another for dessert. There may be a glass, or several of them if it's a formal dinner: one for water, another for the dinner wine, and yet another for a dessert wine. There might also be coffee or tea cups, a small bread plate, a salad plate, even a butter plate. In addition, there will be a napkin, perhaps folded in a certain way. All of these artifacts are part of the ritual of food possession passed on to Americans from European settlers.

While it is true that all of these items are utilitarian, they also help to define our food rituals. The very placement of the implements sends a signal to everyone in the family, silently declaring this meal to be a special event. At formal dinners served in this way, there is even a hierarchy established, with the host as the person who possesses or "owns" the food that will be offered. If it's truly a formal dinner the host or hostess may exert a great many additional controls, such as where people will sit at the table and exactly when they will sit down, literally staking out particular boundaries for each guest.

But formal dinners are not the only ones where the ritual of eating defines specific relationships. Take a moment to reflect on the different signals that are sent by different kinds of place settings and environments. For example, if there are only two place settings with champagne glasses, fine linen napkins and silver, and a small vase of flowers at the center of the table under low lighting, a signal of intimacy would be sent. This is going to be a romantic meal! But if there are six place settings and bright lights, the signal would probably indicate a special group event. Think about other specific place settings and what they signal to those who are to participate in the meal: perhaps a company picnic with uniformed caterers serving from shiny steel food warmers; or a potluck dinner with great pots and trays of food from dozens of different kitchens; or a plastic-wrapped meal on an airplane served on small plastic trays. Let your imagination and your memory entertain these different possibilities and study what part each one plays in your eating experience.

Now focus your attention in a slightly different way, this time on specific ways that food was shared and eaten at your house when you were a child. Take a few minutes to re-live the ritual of food possession as it played out in your past. If this memory brings up emotional content, take the time to be with yourself, and relive those powerful experiences. Record as much as you want in your Food Awareness Journal.

Here's a page from my own Food Awareness Journal:

The stage is now set, on and around the table. . . . and I am impressed with how it indeed resembles a stage set. So, let the play begin! At our family gatherings, my grandmother always announced the beginning of the meal. When we heard her voice, everyone stopped what they were doing and came to the table, where they seated themselves in a familiar order, always in the same chairs. With everyone seated, large plates of food were brought from the kitchen by my grandmother, my mother, and sometimes my sister, too.

As I look back on it, the grand entrance of the food seemed almost like the trumpets announcing the king's entrance in a Shakespearean play, or the tune "Hail To The Chief" announcing the arrival of the President of the United States. It was a triumphant moment—at this point it is clear that the food is the possession of my grandmother and anyone else who had a hand in preparing it. This gift from my grand-

mother to everyone was acknowledged through proper compliments from the guests: "Mm-m-m. It smells so good! Look at that! It's beautiful!"

Grandmother bows her head, a little embarrassed by this sudden display of attention. She modestly waves us away, dismissing our compliments as unimportant, though everyone knows that they are not, that not until the compliments are complete will she announce, "Well, everybody get started before the food gets cold." As much as we might take all of this for granted, it was part of the ritual of food possession at her house and part of our food experience.

Recalling the powerful influence of ritual in these family gatherings, I cannot help but think of a pride of lions at a kill in Africa. In fact, to express how I really felt at those times, I'd call this moment when the food was on the table and the eaters were gathered around "dividing the kill," though at my grandmother's house, thanks to the rituals and artifacts employed, anxiety about who will eat was fairly well democratized, removing the need for serious competition that separates the strong animals from the weak in the wild. Nevertheless, receiving food is a serious business. At the base of it we recognize that the quest for food is a life and death matter. Our rituals assure us that there will be enough, and that we need not fight each other at every meal to eat and stay alive. . . . . .

Although our food rituals mask the immediate recognition of our primal needs, there is a part of each one of us that knows these needs exist. None of us are immune to the basic fact that without food we will not survive.

Our food rituals ensure that there will be enough, and that we need not fight each other at every meal to eat and stay alive.

LEARNING TO HUNT

In your imagination go into a scene from your food past and look at it in detail. In my case, I see everyone seated at the table again, and a blessing has just been offered. I slow the scene down and notice the expressions on people's faces as the moment for the passing of food arrives. I watch the people's eyes. They are *surveying the kill*. Consciously or unconsciously as the plates of food are passed, everyone is asking themselves, how much of this food is for me? Which foods look the most inviting or delicious to me? Which foods will I take or avoid? In this instant, everyone at the table is participating in a powerful but primitive ritual—*the hunt*.

ONE BOWL

We hunt with our eyes, exploring what we can safely claim for ourselves.

EXERCISE:

> The next time you sit down to eat with your family or friends, take a moment before the food is served to take part in the hunt. Here's how. The hunt begins when everyone is seated and the food is on the table, and it ends when everyone has served their plates and are ready to begin eating. During this period, watch the other people. Do their eyes stare at the food, wandering over each dish? Do they avoid looking at the food, and focus inward instead? How do the people you regularly eat with practice the hunt? Most adults hunt with their eyes, while children may hunt with their fingers. Describe what you discover about hunting in your Food Awareness Journal.

EAT IN COURSES

With these food explorations completed, it's time to get down to the basics: how you will incorporate the One Bowl method into your everyday life. To review briefly: you've gotten your bowl, you have reflected on the importance of your daily food rituals, and also thought about some of the eating rituals you presently engage in. In addition, you have begun recording your insights in your Food Awareness Journal.

Meanwhile, you've become comfortable with the bowl you've chosen. Now it's time to begin eating from your bowl every meal that you eat at home. During this initial period you will eat the same foods as you always do, just putting them into your bowl instead of a plate. Although you may feel uncomfortable eating from a bowl at first, really this is only a small change. To solve the problems caused by your bowl's small size, you should place only one food into the bowl at a time. In other words, you will eat in courses.

If previously you ate three to five different foods at a meal, all arranged on your plate next to each other, now you will fill your bowl three to five times in succession, each bowlful containing a different food. You will find that it takes you a bit longer to eat this way, but the benefit is that you will become more aware of the taste of each food. You are now eating with your family or friends, and eating the same foods as they do, at the table with them, but unlike them, you are eating in courses. After all, you would pay good money to eat in courses at a fancy French restaurant, so you may as well enjoy it!

If you don't like mixing the remnants of foods in your bowl, you

ONE BOWL

have the option of washing your bowl between courses. You may also notice that by eating from a bowl, one food at a time, your eating rhythm is different from that of family or friends who eat from their plates at the same table. You are eating more slowly than they are. Refilling the bowl between courses is more leisurely.

Let yourself become comfortable eating this way—from your bowl, in courses. While you will find yourself taking more time to eat, you will also be pleasantly surprised to discover how satisfying the One Bowl method of eating can be. After a meal, each food will linger more distinctly in your memory, and eating will have been a series of gifts, linked together by your bowl.

After a meal, each food will linger
more distinctly in your memory,
and eating will have been a series
of gifts, linked together by your bowl.

EXERCISE:

The purpose of this exercise is to explore what values you place on food— in the broadest sense, exploring how certain foods appeal to you, and how you feel if you waste some food.

Go into your kitchen and, holding your bowl as you would if you were eating, survey the different foods that you might ordinarily eat when you are eating from a regular dinner plate. This is just a practice session, so there is no need to actually eat anything. Just choose a food, figure out how to fit it into your bowl, look at it, smell it, then remove it. If you think of foods you like to eat but that are not in your kitchen at this time, repeat this process in your imagination, figuring out how those foods, too, might fit into your bowl.

As you go through the cupboards or your refrigerator, place foods you might ordinarily eat into your bowl, look at them, smell them, and then discard them. That's right, actually throw the food away. Pay attention to any thoughts or feelings that arise during this process. Does this feel wasteful? Do you feel guilty? Throw away two or three different servings of food and try to identify any feelings of discomfort you experience. Record your observations in your Food Awareness Journal.

As more and more people are beginning to understand, food is a sacred substance. To discard perfectly good food may challenge some deep-seated feelings and beliefs you have. Did your mother always remind you of the starving people in the world, people who would love to have the food you refused to eat when you were a child? Wasting food is sacrilegious, a part of you might say. Record your thoughts and feelings about this issue in your Journal. If your spouse or a friend is practicing the One Bowl method along with you, discuss these issues with them and later record your conversations in your Food Awareness Journal.

At this point in your food exploration journey, you should be carrying out the first part of the One Bowl method. During each meal that you eat at home, you continue all your old familiar eating habits, except for three small changes:

1. You eat only from your bowl.
2. You claim the entire table of "free food" still in the serving dishes as possible food choices.
3. You eat in courses, filling your bowl with only one food at a time and eating that food until it is gone.

Within a few days, you should begin to feel at home eating from your bowl, and familiar with how you like to eat from it. New food habits will be forming. Take your time getting acquainted with these changes in your eating patterns. I've noticed that people who regularly eat alone adjust to One Bowl eating faster than those who mostly eat with a family or a group of friends. If you do regularly eat with others, remember that you have to give these other people time to adjust to your One Bowl eating method, too, and you may want to explain the process to them.

There's a good chance that by now you have begun to wonder how you are going to eat according to the One Bowl method when eating at school, at work, in a restaurant, or at someone else's home. The answer is simple: Don't try to. Confine your One Bowl eating entirely to your own living space. When you eat away from home, eat from a plate just like everyone else does. Later, we will explore new ways to handle the special problems incurred by eating out.

EAT ALONE

After you feel comfortable eating in courses—one food at a time from your bowl—the next step is to begin eating alone. You will maintain your same diet of foods as before, eating from your bowl, in courses. But now eat those foods alone. Pick a favorite room or other area of your living space and sit there alone with your bowl. Make yourself comfortable in all the ways you know you like. Then hold your bowl in your hand and eat. You might choose to eat in bed, on your back porch, up in your favorite tree, or in a special corner of the living room. Take time to choose a place that really appeals to you, where you can enjoy a sense of solitude and peace that allows you to focus inwardly.

Fill your bowl and eat one course in this special place. When you are ready to fill your bowl again, simply get up, leave your special place, get more food in your bowl, and return. Hold the bowl in your hand and eat from it.

You do not need to always eat in the same place, but do always eat in a place you like, one where you can eat in solitude. While you are eating, avoid diversions such as watching television, reading a book, taking care of business for home or school, or otherwise distracting yourself. Just quietly enjoy the pleasure of eating. Put your attention on the food in your possession, relax and enjoy the sensations of taste, and of chewing and swallowing. Eat standing, sitting, or lying down—whatever pleases you. During this special time, let eating become a luxury in your life. Bask in this luxury.

You may find this one part of the One Bowl method the most difficult part to accept. If the idea of eating alone makes you feel uncomfortable, ask yourself why. However, it is important that you carry out this part of the One Bowl method, for this reason: Eating alone is the only way you can really begin to become aware of the subtle but normal sensations of food assimilation occurring within you. Eating alone is the key to learning how to hear your food symphony. It is the only way to begin to understand the natural, inner language of eating.

> *Eating alone is the key to learning how to hear your food symphony.*

When you eat your meals with other people your attention is on them or on your relationships to them, on the problems they have, or the problems you have, on experiences you've had during the day that you want to share with them—a million different things. But it's not on the experience of eating. Also, the tempo and rhythm of your eating pattern—how fast or slow you eat—is dramatically affected when you eat with other people. It is not just that they eat faster or slower than you do, but that a group of people, or even two people, will set up their own collective rhythm which may or may not be in harmony with your own.

Later, after you have become thoroughly familiar with your food symphony—your own inner rhythms and language of eating—it will be possible to eat with others and not lose touch with your own experience. But for now, while you are learning, I highly recommend eating alone.

While you are changing your way of eating to the One Bowl method, it's particularly important to find a wonderful place to eat and to do so in a totally conscious way. Maybe it's somewhere you have never eaten before. Maybe it will be somewhere you will never eat again. The only requirement is that it be just the most wonderful place to eat you can find right at this moment. What are your boundaries for this exploration? Allow yourself to wander and roam in this quest—anywhere in the house and if you have a yard, anywhere in your yard. Once you have found that most wonderful spot, stand, sit, or lie down to enjoy your bowl of food.

After you have finished eating, name out to yourself or write down in your Food Awareness Journal a list of the qualities that describe your chosen eating place. Is it open, secluded, noisy, quiet, indoors or outdoors, warm or cool, colorful or drab, beautiful or interesting, with living plants or among manmade things? I'm sure you can add to this list of characteristics.

Naturally, if you live with other people, when you begin to eat alone everyone will have to make some adjustments. If you are the person who regularly prepares food for family members or friends, then you should continue to prepare their food just as you have before. Cook the food, put it on the table, announce the meal, then fill your bowl with your first course. After your family or friends are seated at the table excuse yourself, find your special eating place, and eat alone. Of course, let your family or friends know what you are doing and why so that the other members won't take your absence as an affront.

If another person regularly prepares food for you, when the food arrives at the table, fill your bowl with your first course, then excuse yourself and take your food away from the table to eat alone. It may not seem like it at first, but most people have less trouble establishing this new eating routine than you might think.

If mealtimes are the only times you have to visit with your family members or friends, you may feel that you must choose between your family and using the One Bowl method. However, there are other alternatives. For one thing, you could arrange to eat before or after everyone else eats and sit at the table with them while they are eating. This way you could satisfy your own food needs, as outlined by One Bowl, and still maintain the social connections with your family.

When my kids were young, our family experimented with a

number of different eating patterns. In fact we dispensed with organized meals altogether for a few months. In other words, everyone in the family ate One Bowl. This worked pretty well, but we had to figure out other ways to be social together. And it was interesting to walk around the house at different times of the day to find someone quietly eating, curled up on a sofa in the living room! But soon, everyone got used to it. The kids liked the freedom this new style of eating gave them. And Eugenia and I had to get over her trepidation that the kids would only eat a narrow range of foods. Actually, they did not! More on this later.

However, I do not recommend this step unless you and your family are naturally moved to it. In other words, don't force solitary eating on anyone! Everyone must find their own special way of handling this problem. Be creative! When you develop solutions to this problem that fit everyone in your family, describe them in your Food Awareness Journal.

Note: children often find eating by the One Bowl method a lot of fun. If you feel like it, let them join in. They will like using a bowl if you are using one, and they will love hunting for a good spot to eat it in. Just don't let their playfulness disrupt the seriousness of your own eating exercise.

L et the idea of eating alone launch a new food education period in your life. After you have solved any socialization problems associated with eating the One Bowl way, let the next several weeks or months be a time apart, in which you will focus your attention on your own relationship to food, on what you eat, and on how your body responds to it.

As you proceed, you will see ways to begin re-integrating eating into your social life, and you will gradually do so. Don't worry! You are not permanently isolated from the human race! This is a sort of training period, that's all. It's a temporary retreat, if you will, from your everyday routine in order to better understand yourself and the many roles food plays in your life.

Winifred, one of the "graduates" of the One Bowl method, found after three months that she was able to stay in touch with her food awareness even under the challenging conditions of being the step-mom in a family with four active children. She had learned during the period when she ate alone to stay centered on her bowl and her feelings associated with food. In time, even eating with a regular dinner plate in front of her, surrounded by all the excitement that vari-

ONE BOWL

ous family members brought to the table, she was still able to stay pretty focused on the One Bowl principles she'd learned. Whenever she lost her ability to concentrate in this way, she took a period of several days during which she ate her meals alone and got back in touch with her body's responses and any feelings that arose as she ate. Like Winifred, you can come and go from One Bowl as you like. It will always be there waiting for you, and it will always work.

THE DE-SOCIALIZATION OF FOOD

From the examples we've discussed, it is clear that social conventions surrounding food have a powerful impact on our individual eating experiences. So it should come as no surprise that for most people, concerns about food choices, digestion, comfort with yourself, and body weight are all intimately connected with the socialization of eating. When you begin to eat alone, you may initially feel lonely, bored, cold, depressed, or even not hungry. These feelings can be confusing and uncomfortable at first. Just let them be and pay attention to them. What are your feelings telling you? Hold these feelings as part of the process of changing your relationship to food. Once you accept them in this way, you'll move beyond them.

Once you have established your new One Bowl eating pattern, any challenging feelings you might have had about eating alone will fade away and you will discover new pleasures to replace your old familiar ones. People have usually reported feeling energized, liberated, and relieved to eat alone in the One Bowl way, even if it's only one meal a day.

Whether your response is to feel loneliness or relief when you start eating alone, it is a testimony to the power of the socialization of food in our lives. And you may not experience loneliness or relief, but rather, something completely unique. And that's fine, too. The point is that whatever feelings come up for you will be your truth which you will want to respect and work with.

Once you have settled into the routine of eating alone, the amount and kind of food you will eat will change in some way. You'll discover for example, that whenever you are with other people you eat certain foods in a particular way simply to please them, or to avoid offending them. For example, you might have eaten fish on Friday nights for years, but discover once you are eating alone that you really don't like fish that much. Or, you might never lick your fingers when eating with other people, but find yourself doing it with great delight when you eat alone.

The harder it is for you to accept the idea of eating alone, the

ONE BOWL

more distinctly changed your way of eating is likely to become once you regularly pursue solitary One Bowl eating. Your resistance to making this change may be an indication of just how much you really need it. Some part of you might be clinging to a former food event structure for fear that, if you give it up, something or someone important will be lost. But once this change to solitary eating is made, you may discover that much more has been gained than lost. If you have strong feelings like this, you may be at that point in your food awareness exploration in which you find yourself standing on the edge of a precipice. If you look down it is scary. And the next step in your journey requires a little jump to clear the fall that lies ahead. But once you jump and land safely on the other side, all will be well. You will be stronger for having taken the dare.

The harder it is for you to accept the idea of eating alone, the more distinctly changed your way of eating is likely to become once you pursue One Bowl eating.

Since you may find this part of the One Bowl method—the desocialization of food—the greatest hurdle you will face, go slow.

There are no time pressures or limits here. Each time you eat at home, eat whatever you wish, and eat as much of it as you wish. And try to eat alone.

At this point, you are only trying to make changes in the *way* you eat. You are still eating the same foods—whatever you choose. The main thing you are doing at this point is isolating food distractions in your life: seeking a quiet space, entering it, closing the door, and being with your private feelings around food and eating.

I recall one woman, Lydia, who wrote me a letter a couple months after starting the One Bowl method. This is what she said:

> *I have always hated eating alone and doing it voluntarily for your program seemed absurd the first few times I did it. I felt deprived and really very sad the first times I tried to eat this way. But as per your suggestions, I stayed with the plan you described and slowly things opened up for me. I know the most important insight for me, that came early on in this experiment, was that I always felt guilty when I ate alone.*
>
> *Then one day, I remembered that whenever I misbehaved at the supper table as a child, my mother sent me to my room and wouldn't let me come out until I had promised to eat everything on my plate. A clean plate was literally my passport back into Mom's good graces. I'd completely forgotten all this and when I finally remembered it, I*

noticed a big switch happening in my attitudes about solo eating. Now
I look forward to my time alone and I no longer feel the pressures of
having to act like an adult at the table or clean my plate.

Oh, I can still hear my mother's words, scolding me for not hold-
ing my fork just right or talking too loud or putting an elbow on the
table, but now it just amuses me and I don't put that kind of pressure
on myself around eating. I have begun to lose weight—but the inner
weight that is gone now is a whole ton—and that's what I want to
thank you for.

Responses like Lydia's are perfectly natural. You may never have
realized before that social eating changes your body's response to
food. Therefore, give yourself time to discover if what I am saying
is true for you. Most people, after a week spent eating alone, find
that they prefer it to social eating most of the time because of the
quiet personal pleasure it brings.

If they are not doing the One Bowl method with you, your
mate, partner, or friend might object to this idea. Obviously,
whenever you choose to eat alone, they are forced to eat alone
whether they want to or not. If this becomes an issue, by all means
sit with them when they eat! Visit with them, but eat before or
after they do. Share the One Bowl ideas with them and try to work
out a common agreement before you start.

ONE BOWL

Keep in mind that most societies put a great deal of emphasis on the socialization of food. Take the time you need to work out the problems of de-socialization that you have, proceeding further only when you are comfortably eating alone and enjoying it.

FEELING FULL

When you have developed your One Bowl eating practice this far, you will have made many changes in your former eating patterns. You still eat your normal diet of foods, but from a bowl. You eat in courses, and you eat alone. No longer do you talk to other people, watch TV, talk on the phone, read, do homework, or go over the bills. You are sitting in your favorite eating place, alone, feeling calm and relaxed, and enjoying your food.

With this much accomplished, it's time to move to the next step, which is learning to focus on recognizing when to stop eating. How do you know when to stop?

TAKING ONE BITE

EXERCISE:

The next time you feel hungry, sit in your favorite eating place with a desirable food in your bowl. Eat calmly.

Pay attention to the wonderful taste and textures of each bite you take. How would you describe the taste, the texture? In your Food Awareness Journal, list the food or foods you are now eating. If you have a sandwich, list the sandwich and then all of its component parts. Do the same for any other combination food you might be eating, such as a casserole. If you don't know all of the ingredients, guess.

The first time I did this exercise, I carefully recorded how each bite of food I ate tasted. I labeled them bite 1, bite 2, and so forth in my Journal. Do this, noting any changes you experience as you proceed from your first bite to the last. This may seem arduous at first but do it and see what happens. I know that for most people this process opens their minds, their taste buds, and their whole body to new food experiences.

After you swallow each bite, see what sensations you can feel as the food passes down into your body. Record any noteworthy sensations. Repeat this exercise again later. How was it different, or not different, from the other days?

As you continue eating, notice whether your sense of being hungry is changing. If it is changing, note and record these changes in your Journal. After you have eaten more than one half of the food in your bowl, begin to pay attention to whether you can notice the sensation of becoming full as you eat. If you can, record what that sensation feels like.

Now continue eating until you definitely begin to feel full. However, try to stop eating the very moment you first feel satisfied. Just sit with yourself and enjoy the sensation for a while. Try to note the exact moment you began to feel full. Could you tell just when that was? How would you describe the sensation we call "full?"

Make notes in your journal about this experiment. Now stand up gently and take your bowl back into the kitchen. Either save or discard the remaining food and wash your bowl. This part of the process is just as important as filling your bowl in the first place, since discarding food and washing your bowl announces to your entire being that you are full and there is no further need to eat. Is

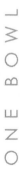

ONE BOWL

7 9

it difficult to stop eating before your bowl is empty? Repeat this exercise on another day. How was it different this time, or not?

At each meal you eat by the One Bowl method, you will be focusing your attention on the food you eat, and on how each bite tastes. You will feel what it's like to chew your food and swallow well. You are probably eating less food now, just because it's easier to tell when you first start to feel full, and as soon as you feel these sensations you stop eating. You probably find eating more satisfying than you had previously and you look forward to eating as a time in which you can relax and truly be with yourself. These changes are simple to describe, but they may be profound in their effect upon your sense of well-being.

After many years spent eating One Bowl, I know that eating is one of the most complex activities I undertake each day, and I am learning to treat it with greater respect. I recognize that eating begins with the first tiny vibrations of hunger inside me—a vibration that grows continually stronger until finally I am set into motion, hunting food. I have come to understand that eating includes deciding what food I want to eat, the way it will be prepared, under what circumstances I will eat it, how fast or slow I

ONE BOWL

will chew and swallow, and the process of digestion and assimilation that goes on without my conscious control during and after the meal. In fact, eating is not truly concluded until my body eliminates as waste the parts of the food it cannot use. All of this is eating; it is my personal food symphony, and I have learned to enjoy it.

In order for me to truly enjoy my meal, many separate elements must come together in harmony. When they do, an inner music fills me and I am truly nourished. When they don't, the result is noise and discomfort.

All of this is eating;
it is my personal food symphony,
and I have learned to enjoy it.

You will gain energy, begin noticing changes in your body and become more comfortable with yourself in general as you learn to increase the harmony in your internal food symphony. It is a simple and natural thing to do once you understand how to do it. In order to develop this understanding, you have to create a time and place in your life in which to focus closely on the food you eat. Everything you have done so far in the One Bowl method brings you to this moment.

When I first reached this point in my food awareness explorations, and was regularly eating one or more meals a day alone, in courses, I soon discovered that by listening to my internal food symphony I began to feel satisfied long before I felt full. In fact, I noticed a kind of structure to my internal food gauge. Once I began eating, my hunger would turn into satisfaction. Then, if I kept eating, my satisfaction would turn into sensations of fullness. If I continued to eat beyond this point, fullness turned into an unpleasant feeling I call stuffed. Full was comforting but stuffed was distinctly uncomfortable. I began to wonder what would happen if I ate less and settled for satisfied instead of full.

So I began to eat just one or two courses at every meal instead of my usual three or four. I did this by stopping eating as soon as I felt satisfied. Formerly I had routinely eaten until I was full (and if I cleaned my plate, until I was stuffed). But now I began to stop with satisfied. After eating only to feel satisfied for a week or so, I noticed that I preferred this sensation over full. One reason was, after each meal I felt light and energized. I never needed to take a nap. This change did cause me to feel hungry sooner than I had before, so I began eating five or six meals a day instead of only three. I did this simply by this means: whenever I felt hungry, I declared it a meal.

Then I noticed that five or six one course meals seemed to distribute my energy better throughout the day. Soon, I preferred to eat one course at a time, and declare this course a meal. From this point forward, I ate some of these meals with my family, and a few with business associates. The majority of my at-home meals were eaten alone, in my special place, with my bowl, one course per meal.

When you feel ready to make this change and try eating to feel satisfied rather than full, simply notice during each meal when that sense of satisfaction occurs, and stop eating at that point. Record in your Journal what you feel about giving up the rest of your food. Record too, how long you go until you feel hungry again. When you do feel hungry, simply declare it a meal and eat again. Record how many meals you eat each day for a week, and whether you prefer satisfied or full, or even stuffed.

Soon I preferred to eat one course at a time, and declare this course a meal.

Once you have reached this stage in the One Bowl method, you are eating most of your meals from your bowl, alone, one course at a meal. Take all the time you need to accommodate these changes to your mind, your body, and your family and friends' needs.

When you feel comfortable with this new form of eating, you will be ready to explore the various foods you eat, to find out which ones are in harmony with your body and which are discordant, creating upset (even digestive upset) and surplus energy (stored as fat). Once you can feel the sensations of discomfort or upset within you that are caused by eating a certain food, then you can choose whether you want to continue eating that food.

On the other hand, when you can feel the sensations of harmony and energy brought to you by a food, you may want to choose to eat foods like that one more often. The more you substitute harmonious foods for those that cause you discomfort, the more completely your body can use that food and the less it has to store as fat. Here's how this works:

ONE BOWL

1. *You will be able to feel more comfortable in your body by decreasing your consumption of disruptive foods and increasing your consumption of harmonious ones.* This first principle is the key to the One Bowl method. However, in order for it to be effective, you must apply it along with four other principles.

2. *Eat whenever you are hungry, as often as you are hungry, but stop eating the minute your hunger ceases.* I never deprive myself of any food I want, or let myself go hungry, but I always stop eating as soon as the sensation of hunger fades. This will be before I feel really full, or stuffed, so I never overeat. But I always feel satisfied.

3. *In the beginning, eat only one food at each meal.* Over time, this has been my preferred way of eating, but this does not mean that everyone should eat this way. Whenever I eat more than one food, I do so in courses. But nine-tenths of my meals are now single-course meals. I eat one food and when hunger ceases I usually feel satisfied and do not refill my bowl.

4. *When you get hungry, make a search to find just the right food that you most want to eat at that particular moment.* Recognize that different moods on different days will

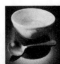

bring the desire for many different foods. Consider *hunting food* an important part of your daily life, and give time to it. . . . all the time you need.

The same food prepared in different ways will have strikingly different effects on your organism. I have found, in general, that foods prepared with seasonings and spices or by frying, tend to be less harmonious for me than the same foods prepared plainly and eaten alone. But this may not be true for you. Many people find certain combinations of foods that work together beautifully for them. If I really enjoy a food that is disruptive to me, I change the manner of its preparation until I have made it more harmonious. In this way I can follow principle five.

5. *I never have to abandon eating any food I like.* People's tastes and responses to food vary enormously. You may find highly spiced foods, or raw foods, or boiled foods, or whatever, more harmonious than I do. One Bowl eating gives you the opportunity to discover what your own individual organism really wants to eat at every meal. Honor your being by finding and eating that perfect food.

I did not apply these five principles to my eating method overnight; they evolved gradually over a period of many months. I actually began by applying only the second and third principles. Each time I felt hungry, I declared it a meal and ate from my bowl until I was no longer hungry. And I ate only one food at each meal. In this way I pretty much continued my former selection of foods, eating just about whatever my family ate. And I always felt satisfied. How did I do this? By eating whenever I felt hungry, and stopping the moment I felt full. Using this method, I never overate. Sometimes I would eat three meals during a day, just as the other people did, and sometimes I would eat more— occasionally up to six or even seven small meals in a single day.

EATING OFF THE CLOCK

Eating off the clock means eating only when you feel hungry, not just when the clock tells you it's time to eat. Can you let yourself eat whenever you feel hungry? Most people eat by the

ONE BOWL

clock. Up in the morning, 7:00 A.M., must be breakfast. Whistle blows, it's noon so it must be lunch time. And so forth. Welcome to the regulated life—human lives controlled by expedient outside factors— challenging the inner harmony of individual food needs!

This is modern life. Actually it has been a habit of American life since the advent of mass production and the assembly line. After all, it's argued, you can't run an efficient factory if people are going to stop and take breaks any time they wish just because their stomachs are growling! In this country, we take our eating cues from machines!

In southern Europe people tend to close up their shops and take long lunches, which often includes a siesta. They open for business again in the mid-afternoon and work late. Such a scheme may fit the body's natural needs more harmoniously than do the customs of American society, which seems more driven by financial profit than human satisfaction. The line "I Can't Get No Satisfaction," from the song "Satisfaction," would probably not be sung or even imagined in other, more "primitive" societies whose daily activities are determined more by the movements of the sun in the sky and the physical and spiritual messages that come from within.

EXERCISE:

In this exercise you'll be exploring what it would be like to pay more attention to what's going on inside you than what a clock or other external signal is telling you.

Wake up in the morning on a day when you have some free time. Maybe it's your day off. Now, paying attention to your inner food sensations, notice when you first begin to feel hungry. Is it upon waking? Upon rising from the bed? Is it only after you have showered and dressed? Or is it only later, at mid-morning? Eugenia never seems to actually feel hungry until about two in the afternoon while I usually feel starved within a half-hour of rising.

When you actually feel hungry, eat. Try to note whether your hunger has been conditioned to the clock, or to a particular period of the day, or by some other business or personal patterns in your life. In other words, is your hunger/food cycle habitualized, or are you pretty free and open about when you eat? Whatever it is, don't judge it; just notice and record what you find in your Food Awareness Journal. If your life situation allows you to eat whenever you wish for every meal, do you? Or are you voluntarily eating on the clock?

On another day, try this exercise. As twelve noon approaches, pay attention to your inner sensations. Do

ONE BOWL

89

you automatically begin to get hungry? Or could it be that you only begin to feel the sensation of hunger because other people are beginning to talk about food, or are preparing and eating it? Record these discoveries in your Journal.

I know that there are many jobs which require you to eat beforehand in order to get to work. Sometimes you might even have to eat at a specific time, whether you are hungry or not, because due to the nature of your work you might not otherwise get a chance to eat for many hours.

One Bowl is flexible. If you are currently in some work or lifestyle situation which requires you to eat at a specific time, do so. Eat One Bowl wherever possible, then eat by the clock when that is necessary. As you come to fully appreciate the personal benefits of eating off the clock, you will find a new way to make changes in your work or lifestyle situation. Be patient and be optimistic! Follow One Bowl as best you can and watch—things will improve!

Try the following exercise for one week: Each day, keep a log in your Journal of every meal you eat. Simply record: "Breakfast, Monday," then note the time you ate, whether you were actually hungry or were just eating on the clock, and whether you ate alone or socially. Don't try to make conscious changes. Just record these things, watch yourself, and think about it.

LEN AND LILLIAN PEARSON

During the time I was first conducting my One Bowl experiments back in 1973, I had not met Leonard and Lillian Pearson nor heard about their food workshops at the Pearson Institute, even though they were held in Berkeley, California, where I lived. My friend Anne Kent Rush attended their workshop and came to see me one day filled with enthusiasm. She told of spending several hours experimenting with chewing food and how satisfying that simple act was. She told of eating one bean very slowly and completely losing her sense of hunger, as though one small bean could make an entire meal.

She told me about foods that *hum* and foods that *beckon*, and how important it was to search out just the right food you wanted to eat at every meal. For an hour or more Kent told me of these amazing things she had experienced. From this one conversation,

I was fired with new enthusiasm to continue my own food explorations. What Kent was telling me seemed to confirm everything I had discovered up to that point.

In this book, I do not talk about the *psychology of food*, which could be defined as understanding and explaining why people eat as they do, because the Pearsons have pioneered this field in their book *The Psychologist's Eat-Anything Diet* (sadly out of print but you might find this book through Bookfinders.com). Thanks to the Pearson's pioneering work, I could add that important fourth principle to the One Bowl method—to always search for the food I really wanted to eat. I owe the discovery of this fourth principle to the Pearsons.

EATING FROM HUNGER, NOT FROM HABIT

During the initial stages of my food awareness explorations, I would eat from my bowl while sitting with my family, who were having their regular breakfast, lunch, and dinner. My belief at that time was that the social contact during these times was important. However, I also ate several small meals alone, somewhere between one and three more times during the day, whenever I felt hungry. Some meals during each day I ate with my family, and some I ate alone.

*Shift into a pattern of
eating from hunger, and out
of a pattern of eating from habit.*

If I did not feel hungry when my family was eating, I just sat and talked with them. I watched while they ate. This was easy for me to do and they soon grew accustomed to my behavior; we all enjoyed each other's company in the regular way. If you live in a social situation, you might try this method as an easy way to shift into a pattern of eating from hunger, and out of a pattern of eating from habit, while still being reasonably social.

TAKE YOUR TIME

To succeed with the One Bowl method, it must become a natural process for you. Allow yourself the time it will take to adjust gradually and at your own pace to the changes One Bowl brings into your life. Your family and your friends, your job and your habits of life, are essential parts of you. They will shift to accommodate your needs, but perhaps more slowly than you might wish. Someone once told me that life actually changes only at the rate that grass grows, and I believe that this is true. Change moves slowly but small changes now will lead to very large ones

ONE BOWL

9 3

later. Have confidence that if the One Bowl method contains any truth for you, time will bear it out. There is nothing to hurry. You can relax.

Life actually changes
only at the rate that grass grows.
Tarbis Hamsley, unpublished work

LEARNING THE SIGNALS

I said earlier that the key to the One Bowl method lies in your ability to distinguish disruptive foods from harmonious ones, and in your decision to eat more of the latter. Once you can clearly feel a variety of sensations from the different foods you eat, the idea of what's harmonious and what's not quickly becomes clear, and conscious choices about what to eat soon follow. It's simple. We eat what's pleasant and avoid what's not. And once you begin paying attention to your inner food symphony, some formerly pleasant "head" foods may no longer please your body.

When you have begun to eat only one food at each meal, and are eating these meals from your body's signals of hunger instead of from habit or from the clock, you are well on your way to mastering the primary logic of the One Bowl method.

ONE BOWL

W hat is hunger, anyway? My dictionary defines it as a strong or compelling desire for food, or the state of weakness that is caused by a lack of food. This is a state everyone is familiar with, but do we understand it? Is there more to be learned about hunger? Is hunger always and only about food?

For a moment, let's explore this question: What inside of you is hungry for what? Record your answer(s) in your Food Awareness Journal.

EXERCISE:

The purpose of this exercise is to explore exactly what it means to you to feel hungry. The next time you feel hungry, ask yourself: where in your body do you feel this sensation? In your mouth? In your throat? In your stomach? In your mind? In your heart? In more than one place?

Sit in your favorite eating place for a minute and feel the sensation you call hunger singing within you. To me, hunger is like a little beacon, sending me a message

ONE BOWL

and guiding me to make certain life choices. Hunger can stop me in my tracks, disrupt my plans, and temporarily take over my life. What exactly is the sensation you call hunger? Is it continuous? Intermittent? Strong? Weak? Pleasant? Unpleasant? In your Journal, write down a list of the qualities you experience by which you know that you are hungry. Try to capture your sensations of hunger accurately in words.

I suggest that you conduct this hunger exercise before each meal for a few days until your hunger sensations are thoroughly familiar to you. Just allow yourself to feel the sensations you call hunger. At different times they may emanate from different parts of your organism according to your mood, vary as a result of your work or physical activities, time of day, general health, and so forth. These sensations will not always be of the same intensity or quality. To become fully aware of them, don't judge them; just feel them, contemplate them, and describe your experiences in your Food Awareness Journal.

If food is our nourishment, then the symbolic definition of food might be that it represents the mother. Food nourishes us, protects us, and sustains our lives, roles initially carried out by our mothers. If your real mother was not very nurturing to you as a child, you might now, as an adult, have a strong or even inappropriate craving for food as a way to get the essential nourishment that you missed in your early developmental years.

This is a psychological way of saying that I can crave something which I legitimately need, and which I try to satisfy by eating food, but which is really a need belonging to other parts of my organism than my stomach. I might overeat because I am trying to fill an emotional need. The sensation of feeling full in my stomach might temporarily ameliorate my emotional craving, but it does not satisfy the real need I'm trying to fill, so I eat more. Over time I perhaps gain weight or experience other forms of discomfort, whether physical, emotional, or spiritual, yet my eating never really satisfies me. Something in me is calling out to be fulfilled.

If you find yourself unable to follow the One Bowl method, I suggest that you take a look at the symbolic nature of your hunger.

ONE BOWL

9 7

A good way to do this is to read and work with *The Anxiety and Phobia Workbook*, by Edmund Bourne. This book is available from Amazon.com, or any well-stocked bookstore.

EXERCISE:

The purpose of this exercise is to get in touch with the essential non-food needs that you might be trying to satisfy by eating. Look at and smell the food you have put into your bowl. Now that you have chosen it, does it seem to be exactly the food you most want to eat right now? Is it the perfect food? If not, put that food aside and fill your bowl with something that promises greater satisfaction.

If only one part of your being wants the food; which part is it? Your mind? For example, did you choose a food because you thought it would be healthy for you? Did your emotional state choose it because it promised to bring comfort? Or energy? Did your stomach choose that food, or your head? Did you feel uncomfortably hungry and just want something to temporarily allay your feelings?

If it seems as though all the parts of you really want to eat this food, and you can feel yourself responding to

O N E   B O W L

the food with enthusiasm, just let yourself bask in the sensations of *food anticipation* for a moment. Hold off from eating, and just contemplate your desire. This is raw hunger. Explore what it is like for you. Record any discoveries in your Journal.

The more frequently you do this exercise before you eat, the more intensely familiar the sensation of desire will become to you, and the more finely honed your ability to choose the right food will be. Of course, these sensations will vary among foods and as your energy and moods differ from one day to the next. See if, over a period of time, you can detect a pattern to all these different sensations, from responding to a food only because you think it is good for you, to responding because your whole body tells you "I want that now!" In your Food Awareness Journal, write down the results you discover.

FOOD THAT HUMS

During any visit to a kitchen pantry, a family or restaurant buffet, or even while scanning a menu, many foods may call out to you at once. Any food that calls to you, if eaten, will likely produce deep satisfaction. Your organism will resonate to it. When I resonate to a food, I sometimes say (thanks to the Pearsons) that the food "hums."

A food that hums is a very pleasing event; I can look forward to eating it because I can just feel in advance that it will be very satisfying to me. In my family, people can be heard to declare, "Nothing hums today," as a way of describing their inability to find a food they really want to eat. Or they say something like, "I'm going to eat a banana—it really hums." Humming foods have entered my family's vocabulary big time.

The musical quality of humming seems to be an appropriate label to describe the experience I feel upon locating the perfect food for any moment. If a food is just right, we are vibrating together—that food and I. This quality of humming speaks to the utterly earthy connection that exists between a person and their food. Do you try to eat what hums?

The next time you feel hungry, hunt for a food that hums. Go to your happy hunting grounds—your kitchen, refrigerator, grocery store, or restaurant—wherever it is, and begin the hunt. How does one find that perfect food? There is nothing to explain. Just go hunting and you will soon discover the answer. Look over the foods you see. Hold them in your hand. Imagine eating them.

Don't stop until you have located at least one humming food.
Record your hunting and humming discoveries in your Journal.

> When I resonate to a food,
> I usually say that the food "hums."

EXERCISE:

Take one bite of your food, and chew it thoroughly. How does it feel to your tongue, teeth, cheeks? Note textures, tastes, and the interactions between all the various parts of your mouth that become involved as you chew. As you chew, what, if anything, is happening to your feeling of hunger? Is this food satisfying your hunger? Is it increasing your hunger? Is it making you crave some other food? How do your teeth feel? What does your tongue think about this food? Can you hold a short dialogue with your tongue, asking if it enjoys what you are eating?

Focus all your attention on chewing for a moment.

ONE BOWL

Enjoy chewing one bite of food for as long as you like. Does it stay enjoyable to chew? What causes you to swallow it? Write down what you discover about chewing in your Food Awareness Journal.

LEARNING TO SWALLOW

EXERCISE:

The purpose of this exercise is to become acquainted with sensations in your body after you have chewed your food. Take a bite of food. Can you feel it in the back of your mouth? In your throat? In your esophagus? In your stomach?

Pay attention to what is happening in your body as you swallow that bite. Try to follow your bite as it settles into your stomach. For how long after you swallow it can you feel that bite moving inside you?

After swallowing, ask yourself why you swallowed. Was the food no longer tasty? Were you bored? Did you get impatient with the exercise and just want to get on with your eating? If you only swallowed the food

ONE BOWL

because you were trying to do everything these instructions suggested, treat the next bite of food differently. Don't swallow it until you are good and ready to swallow it, then swallow and ask yourself why.

Write down what you have discovered in your Food Awareness Journal. While you did this swallowing exercise were you impatient? Restless? Playful? Angry? Judgmental? Serene? Record these reactions, too.

VISUALIZE ONE BITE OF FOOD

EXERCISE:

The purpose of this exercise is to increase your awareness of the process of a single bite of food going down into your stomach and into your system. Each bite of food is like a deep-sea diving expedition. You drop something important over the side—a sounding instrument. Now, for how long can you feel it descending down inside you?

Imagine that you have just put your favorite food into your bowl and are eating it. See this food in your

ONE BOWL

mind's eye. You can describe it in words in your Journal, or draw a picture of it.

Focus on one imaginary bite of it. Imagine chewing, tasting, swallowing, and then following it down into your stomach. After swallowing this imaginary bite of food, has there been any change in your feelings of hunger? What does the rest of your body feel now? Has it changed? What about your mood? What about your energy? Are you more relaxed? Less relaxed? Is your breathing relaxed? Is your body comfortable?

Repeat this simple, silent procedure for eating a bite of imaginary food before you begin each meal over the next few days. By doing this, you will gain a new familiarity with the food you eat, and in addition, collect valuable information about your body's inner feelings toward different foods.

After eating one imaginary bite, begin eating your real food in this same way. Take a bite, then close your eyes and visualize the food you are eating in your mind's eye. Watch yourself chew, taste, and swallow it, then follow that bite all the way down into your stomach. What did you discover from this exercise? You may be surprised at how well you can track food after you swallow it.

You may notice new attributes about the food you have been eating. Some favorite foods may suddenly not taste so good, while others may taste better than you ever expected. You may also find that the first few bites of some favorite foods will produce a noticeably positive or negative effect in your stomach, while others seem to have little effect, even a half hour after eating.

And you may find that some of your favorite foods actually cause digestive discomfort, in the form of mild pain, burping, gas, or heartburn. Record these discoveries in your Journal.

Each bite of food is like a deep sea diving expedition. You drop something important over the side—a sounding instrument. Now, for how long can you feel it descending inside you?

You may have discovered that this exercise has helped to make you more aware of the total sensations occurring in your body as you eat. This is your food symphony at work. It plays you a tune composed of various bodily sensations. Many of these sensations will be more subtle than a strong sensation such as digestive upset.

Instead, they are the normal sensations that accompany eating, such as motion, temperature change, energy change, satisfaction, or tranquility.

As you try to focus on what is happening to each bite of food you swallow, see whether you can actually experience these kinds of subtle sensations. Here's a possible list.

EMPTINESS

An area of emptiness

A feeling of weight, heaviness or a heavy area

Weight moving from one place to another

Weight turning over and over

Weight that flows like liquid

Weight suddenly released, then emptiness

PRESSURE

Pressure building up

Pressure decreasing

Pressure suddenly released

Pressure changing

Pressure moving from one place to another

Pressure changing as a result of weight changes

ONE BOWL

TEMPERATURE

A food swallowed that feels warm

A food swallowed that feels cold

A body area beginning to feel warm

A body area beginning to feel cold

A body area changing temperature

Temperature changes as a result of pressure changes

Temperature changes as a result of weight changes

MOVEMENT

A slow movement

A rhythmical, repetitive movement

A rapid, vibratory movement

A movement that grows

A movement that diminishes

A movement as a result of pressure changes

A movement as a result of weight changes

A movement as a result of temperature changes

Movements of body organs

A change in intensity of movement of an organ

A muscle you tighten

A muscle you tighten as a result of changes in

    weight, pressure, temperature or movement

ONE BOWL

SOUND

An area of sound

A continuous, gurgling sound

A sharp, one-time sound

A sound that begins, changes, or ends as a result of
changes in any of the above characteristics

In your Food Awareness Journal, record a short list of the sensations you have experienced from eating one bite of food. It might or might not include any of the above.

PROPRIOCEPTIVE SIGNALS

As you read through the list, you will probably realize right away that you recognize these sensations, and perhaps other variations and combinations I haven't listed. They are merely those little feelings that always seem to be going on inside your body. Scientists call them "proprioceptive signals." They are not symptoms of any illness, but rather the natural sensations that accompany the experience of living in a human body.

Pay attention to these signals. Consider them special messengers to you, friendly messengers that are constantly sending you information about any food or drink you have ingested. You can become more aware of them whenever you wish, just by paying attention. When you do, you will get signals with every bite of food you take. These signals may come from your mouth, your throat, your stomach, or your intestines—which means anywhere up and down the length of your torso. They may also be associated with your emotional state, or your energy state.

These signals usually begin when you first feel hungry, grow stronger and more varied as you begin to eat, continue strongly for a half hour after eating (sometimes longer), and finally conclude only after you go to the bathroom. This length of time—from the first feeling of hunger, through eating, to elimination—can be considered one complete food cycle. Usually you will begin several food cycles before completely concluding the previous ones, so there are always foods in different stages of different cycles in your body, all sending signals simultaneously.

For our purposes it is enough to become aware of those signals that are strongest immediately before, during, and for a half hour after eating. To be thorough in your Food Awareness Journal, you could write down the sensations you feel after a first bite of imaginary food, then a first bite of real food, then again after the food in your bowl is half eaten, and finally after you have finished your meal.

Let me repeat an important point. All of these proprioceptive signals are a part of your normal digestive and assimilative body processes. They are not signs of illness. All of them come to you in the form of either sensations or feelings, having three general patterns:

1. *The strongest signals are usually more important than the weakest.*
2. *Their intensity and quality changes as you eat* (over a period of time you will see a pattern to these changes).
3. *You can judge the meaning of each signal by how it makes you feel.*

Depending on what these food sensations are, they will definitely affect your general sense of well-being. If you have stomach pains, you feel irritable and unproductive. But when you have eaten well of a food that hums, you will feel buoyant and optimistic. Before eating you may feel slightly nervous, charged, or empty and weak. Afterward you may feel drowsy, relaxed, energized, or contented. A little later you are filled with purpose again. Remember, no two people respond exactly the same way. Record in your Journal how you feel after eating any meal composed of a food that hums for you.

Each time you eat, listen for a minute or two to all the signals you can get from your first bite of food. Then as you eat, notice any changes you feel in your sense of well-being. Since you are eating only one food at a time, you will be able to relate any changes you experience directly to that particular food.

Let's say that you are trying to evaluate the food you have just eaten but you are not sure if it really is harmonious with your body. I have found that the best way to deal with this question is to not worry about it too much. Some foods clearly make me feel good; others clearly do not. Those are easy. Still others seem okay but nothing outstanding or obvious occurred when I ate them. I wasn't really sure about them. So I made this rule: unless or until I decide that a food is definitely upsetting to me, I continue to eat it, though I try to pay closer attention to the eating. Gradually I have developed three criteria to help me evaluate the meaning of the many proprioceptive signals I receive:

1. *Every food I eat affects my mood.* The most harmonious foods either make me feel good about myself or keep

ONE BOWL

111

me feeling good. Foods that leave me feeling worse than before I began to eat, I consider not harmonious, and I avoid them.

2. *Every food I eat changes the available energy I have.* Some foods make me feel drowsy, some sluggish, some charged up. I rate any food according to whether it increases my energy or reduces it.

3. *Every food I eat affects my overall body stability.* Some foods make me feel fat, heavy, bulky, massive, slow. Others make me feel tall, thin, lithe, or fast. Still others make me feel physically out of touch, disconnected, unbalanced, or spacey. These and many similar body sensations, though subtle, are just as real to me as my mood or my energy, and I give them equal attention.

I identify all of these phenomena as intimate parts of myself, and recognize that changes occur in all of them continually. I have found that during the course of a day, by using the One Bowl method, I can easily notice the changes in my mood, my energy, and my body feelings that are produced by the foods I eat.

Though I can always feel a connection between the signals I get while eating and digesting food, and the changes in mood, energy, and body feelings a food produces, this connection is complex, since the possible combinations of signals and feelings are infinite. Therefore it would be impossible to catalog them all. Instead, I just watch the overall patterns.

If, when I eat, the food tastes good, dissipates my hunger, produces no unpleasant inner signals, and does not make me feel irritated or depressed, sluggish or nervous, full or heavy, I consider that I have eaten pretty well. I have learned to look for *level foods*, foods which tend to maintain the good attitude place I am in, which keep my energy flowing steadily, and which do not interrupt my sense of well-being.

> I have found that during the course
> of a day, by using the One Bowl
> method, I can easily notice
> the changes in my mood, my energy,
> and my body feelings that are
> produced by the foods I eat.

BRANCHING OUT

Once you are regularly eating according to the One Bowl method, you are no doubt undergoing changes. You are feeling better physically and mentally. Eating is a more calm and meaningful experience for you. Most probably your body feels different now: you may have more energy, feel lighter, enjoy better moods. Take the time to appreciate these changes. Don't drive yourself too hard. Now that you are confident that the One Bowl method works for you, there's no hurry. Try not to hold yourself within too strict limits. Use One Bowl when it feels right and return to social eating when you must.

But when you do eat One Bowl, branch out. Move away from the foods that are familiar to you and begin to try ones you rarely eat. Many factors combine to limit the range of foods people enjoy, not the least of which are habit and convenience. Most people could easily prepare a wider selection of foods, but choose instead to eat the same ones they especially like over and over again. However, you now have a whole new set of criteria to apply to the foods you eat. *You will no longer judge a food just by its taste in your mouth alone, but by your inner body experience of it as well.* There is a whole world of new possibilities to explore.

When I first reached this point with my discovery of the One Bowl method, I conducted a number of new food experiments for myself, the results of which eventually carried my personal food evolution yet one step further. Here's what I did:

1. *I decided to prepare all my meals myself* (or as many as I reasonably could).

2. *I began to experiment with the foods I would eat at a given time of day*—trying meat or potatoes in the morning, for instance, and eggs or cereal at night. In other words, I decided to subject time-of-day foods to inner body criteria. I discovered what I had suspected—that I had confined myself within narrow limits unnecessarily.

3. *I searched for new foods to eat, ones that I had rarely or never eaten before.*

The result of this intensive exploration, after several months, was to teach me new things about myself, increase my confidence in the way I ate, and widen my food vocabulary, giving me greater variety in my eating experience, while increasing my food pleasure. And since my body weight was one of the issues I was personally dealing with, I was also losing weight!

I began to vary my methods of food preparation. At this time I was eating from my bowl five or six times a day, alone, but I was still eating within the range of my family's traditional diet. I soon found that just by varying the food preparation, I could move into

ONE BOWL

new tastes and new possibilities of harmony with a particular food, even one which had not been great for me in the past.

Then one day I decided to try moving away from eating any combinations of food, such as casseroles and stews. I found that I felt better and could successfully eat the same foods that were in those combination foods when they were prepared separately.

Next, I tried eliminating all cooking oils and traditional spices from my food preparation and later, I tried eliminating all fried foods. Still other times I eliminated all forms of sugar, caffeine, all salt and pepper, all beef or pork. Over a period of time I varied my food preparation in any way I thought of or heard about that sounded good.

Eventually all this exploration led me to my present diet, which includes many of the foods I have used all my life, such as fish or chicken, and zucchini, but which I now prepare more simply than before. I used to fry zucchini; it is my favorite vegetable. But now I wash and grate one whole zucchini into shreds directly into an iron skillet then grill it without any oil or butter, turning occasionally with a spatula. I add ground pepper when that hums, and in a few minutes this wonderful vegetable is ready to eat. It is pure zucchini, and it always makes me a harmonious meal. By the way, my friends love it, too. They all say they never

ONE BOWL

heard of fixing zucchini this way, and much prefer it to the softer boiled or baked casserole varieties.

I recount this part of my adventure to encourage you, when you feel ready, to consider food preparation to be a good way to expand your personal food menu, and to consider this exploration to be part of the One Bowl method, and perhaps make it a natural part of your diet too.

> It makes me feel secure to know that I possess a hunting ground where a wide selection of food is always available.

FOOD HUNTING

Each time I get those first familiar signals of hunger from deep within me, I try to stop what I am doing and head for my happy hunting grounds—the kitchen. Hunting food is an important part of the eating process because it is my expression of food possession. It makes me feel secure to know that I possess a hunting ground where a wide selection of food is always available. I allow myself to enjoy these feelings of the hunt, and I often make

ONE BOWL

a game of them. Yes, at my house wild herds of tofu and other exotic animals are allowed to roam the kitchen!

Once in the kitchen, I go to all the different places food is stored—the refrigerator, the pantry, the cabinets, cupboards, and shelves—and I explore what food is in each one. Then I try to let my sense of possession extend over all these areas. I tell myself, *This is my hunting ground for food.*

I begin a typical hunt by trying to match various foods to my hunger. I do this by handling, fondling, poking, squeezing, smelling, fantasizing, and examining as many foods as it takes to find the one that's just right. I am searching for the food that resonates with me, the food that is just right at this very moment, the food that will hum.

Usually I will hunt for three or four minutes and then make my selection, but there have been times when I remained frustrated for up to a half hour because I couldn't settle on the right food. If, at those times, I gave in to expediency and ate just any food that was handy and quick, usually I would continue to feel frustrated after my meal, not hungry but not satisfied, and in this situation would be tempted to eat again even though I was not hungry. Eating foods that don't hum reinforces eating patterns that contribute to the very discomforts we are trying to remove. That feeling of dissatisfaction with a meal can quickly lead me to overeat, because I eat again before I need to.

"But," you say, "how will I know when I have found the right food?" If you have just "eaten to live" for many years, if you have always eaten food someone else has chosen, prepared, and placed before you, then it may be difficult at first for you to be able to recognize when a food is calling to you. Your hunting instincts may be a bit dulled. All of the One Bowl exercises you have carried out in this book so far are designed to stimulate your natural food sensitivity. How will you know when you have found the right food? You just will. Your body will tell you.

But what if I see a food, and remember that I liked it a week ago—is this my body telling me to eat it? Maybe and maybe not. This could be your head talking, and if you choose that food, you may be leaving your body out of the hunting process. The way to tell for sure is to hold that food for a minute while you continue to search your happy hunting grounds. If no other food calls to you more than the one you are holding, eat it.

If you find yourself hunting in the kitchen and are unable to find any foods that call out to you, or you think that several or many foods are calling to you equally strongly, try this hunting instinct exercise.

The purpose of this exercise is to explore the different ways foods call out to you, and help you learn to read these signals more accurately, so that you will more likely choose foods that really hum to you.

The next time you're hungry, go into your food hunting area. Now scan over all the food you see. If, while you scan, you begin thinking about some food, or some meal you enjoyed in the past, or some food you had been planning to try, delete that food from your mind. Assume that this is only your head talking.

Instead, try to feel how your whole organism responds to each food you see. If you have no feeling for it, pass that food by. If, when you see a food, you have an interest in it, see a spontaneous image of it in your mind, as if out of nowhere, or notice a change in the feelings of hunger somewhere in your body, or in your mood or energy state—even a fairly subtle change—then this food is calling to you, all of you, and not just your head. It is really humming.

Realize that in any given hunting ground, many foods will be calling to you. But in this exercise, you are not seeking that one perfect food to eat. You are just

ONE BOWL

attempting to stimulate your own sensitivity to the fine art of food hunting.

DECLARE A HAPPY HUNTING GROUND

Take the time to declare a happy hunting ground in your house and in your feelings, and hunt there every day. Nurture your happy hunting ground by keeping it stocked with a wide variety of "game." This will make your natural food store shopping more interesting too, because a natural food store is a super-sized happy hunting ground. Treat it as such. Let it stock your personal game preserve with lots of yummy things to eat.

HOW TO HUNT IN THE FOOD STORE

Since I discovered the One Bowl method of eating, food stores have taken on a new meaning for me. No longer is it drudgery to shop. Now I have a new attitude. A visit to the natural food store is a chance to revitalize my happy hunting ground at home—a chance to restock the forests, so to speak. When I have time, I take the opportunity to walk all the aisles in the food store with my food feelers out, searching for whatever foods call to me.

The purpose of this exercise is to learn how to make choices by the One Bowl method when you go to the market to buy food. Go to your favorite natural food store. Without pushing a shopping cart, let's go food hunting. In other words, in this exercise you will not actually buy any food, just locate foods that hum for you. Begin at either end of the store and just walk all the aisles, scanning the shelves as you pass by, looking for whatever foods call to you. You don't believe food in a can or a package can call to you when you're not even hungry? Just try it!

Walk the aisles and scan the shelves; see what jumps out at you. Don't have any preconceived idea in your mind about what foods you will like or what sections of the store to visit. Tell yourself it will be okay if no foods call to you. Tell yourself it will be okay if unknown or unexpected foods call to you. Don't analyze whether you are responding to a certain food or to its package. Just be open to the possibilities. Walk the aisles and scan the food. If you see familiar foods, ones you eat all the time, just smile and wave at them; it is like passing old friends on the street. Then get on with your business.

If possible, take your Food Awareness Journal with you. When a food jumps out at you, pick it up, hold it, feel it, imagine eating it. What do you feel? Write down both the name of the food that calls to you, and your response to it. "Okra. I love it. Makes me feel all warm and slimy," and so forth.

Take as long to walk the aisles as you like. Most people find that when they do this exercise, rather than finding no foods calling to them, they find too many! A good half-hour's food hunt can be exhausting.

If during your food hunt, a food jumps out at you that is not uniformly packaged, say a cheese, which might be packaged in different sizes by weight, look over all the cheese packages of that type. Try to discover if one of these packages or sizes of cheese calls to you more than the other cheeses. This is just an exercise to stimulate your food sensitivity. It's just something to try for fun, to see whether one quantity of a food hums more intensely than any other quantity of that same food. You can most easily carry out this exercise with cheeses, fruits, and vegetables because they are not packaged uniformly the way milk, cereal, and canned foods are.

B ody weight is an American obsession. It is important for that reason, to explore what feeds that obsession and to realize that more than anything else this obsession is a symptom of being out of touch with the inner signals of our bodies and out lives. I have not weighed myself for years. But using the One Bowl method I know when my body weight is right for me and when it is time to pay greater attention to my body's inner wisdom.

There are many reasons that people may be drawn to this book, and concern with weight is just one of them. But given that we are daily inundated with external messages about watching our weight, we would be remiss to ignore the fact that these signals can be confusing. To change your perceptions about these signals, I advise you not to judge your progress with the One Bowl method by what you might read on your bathroom scale. Judge instead by your feelings about yourself. Notice changes in your mood, your energy, or your attitudes. Notice how your body feels, how your clothes fit, and your available energy. Weight loss is always accompanied by other, inner changes because excess weight accumulation is only the end product of incongruent food attitudes, eating patterns, and digestive processes. *It is not the removal of weight so much as changing these processes that is your goal.* I have not met anyone who followed the One Bowl method who didn't lose weight, look better, have more energy, and be happier about themselves in general.

Change your food attitudes and a weight loss will naturally follow. If you judge your success or failure with the One Bowl method by the numbers that come up on a scale, you have missed the point of this book. Judging numbers is an objectivizing process. But remember, you are not an object. The so-called objective measurements are the "scientific fictions" that drive the modern world, but that method of looking at your life will not help you to learn how to decipher and heed the inner wisdom of your body.

It may be convenient for doctors to treat you as an object, but you need not look at yourself that way. Nobody knows more about you than you know about yourself. But you also have to believe you can access this knowledge, and then actively do so. Refusing to view yourself as an object is one powerful way to take back your own power as a unique individual. This is an important part of the One Bowl method. Shifting your view of yourself from an object to a subject will help to bring you to yourself.

In the western world, kids are taught to be objects at an early age. In school, they are constantly tested. Tests are an objectivizing

ONE BOWL

device. Like a mirror, they train people to see themselves from the outside. "I am only as good as my grades." Objectification means devaluing the feelings I have about myself in favor of an outside value system imposed by some measuring device, be it a teacher, a doctor, a researcher, my peer group, or the results of some data on a computer.

When you relinquish your evaluation process to another person or system you begin to lose yourself. When you lose yourself, you are not able to be fully present in your life, and the world around you is robbed of your unique gift. This may be a desirable political end for some people in power but it does not serve you, or the world.

The One Bowl method invites you to de-objectify yourself. It teaches you to look at and honor your own inner processes. Let them be your authority. Learn to experience yourself rather than judging yourself. You are who you are in all of your wonderful contradictory diversity. You are also what you have to work with. It is enough.

When you relinquish your evaluation
process to another person or system
you begin to lose yourself. When you

lose yourself, you are not able to be
fully present in your life, and
the world around you is robbed
of your unique gift.

AVAILABLE ENERGY

I use the word *energy* and the phrase *available energy* in this book since one of the chief functions of the digestive process is the production of energy for the body. However, there can be many physical and psychological factors that can block or tie up this energy, draining it off so that it is not available for your use. Therefore, I speak of *available energy* to acknowledge that our potential supplies of energy are not necessarily available to us at all times. I assume that no matter how much energy I think I have, I could always have more. More harmonious use of foods can produce more energy for your use because your body is capable of using certain foods more efficiently than others. For example, some foods are stored in our fat cells rather than being translated into immediately available energy. As you continue to use the One Bowl method, you will begin to feel that you have more energy, and you will experience other new body sensations as well.

These subtle changes can't necessarily be measured in numbers. They are analog not digital experiences. In this highly technological world, people rush to digitize everything without realizing that human experience is not digital. It is fundamentally analogical, and needs to be honored as such. Once you understand and use your analogical sensations, it will be like evaluating the totality of your life weighing from within.

Understanding complex biochemical nutritional needs, counting calories, and developing a balanced diet were important problems for our parents, who lived in the time of an emerging food culture. These measurements are now the standard medical tools for describing the relationships between what we eat and our metabolism. In America today, food is extremely plentiful; the hunting grounds are filled with more "game" than at any time in human history. Every freeway exit is jammed with restaurants. Every city corner has another fast-food depot.

Given the eating habits that have been fostered by our modern world, it is no surprise that a book like One Bowl would be necessary. In a simpler, slower-paced world, people would have an intuitive understanding of their metabolic needs, based on signals from their bodies that they had learned to decipher very early in their lives. They would not have to learn to follow medically calculated food programs; they could just live their body's metabolism.

CRAVINGS

Don't worry, you will not eat chocolate cake for the rest of your life and gain a thousand pounds!

My experience with the One Bowl method has convinced me that when your body really wants a particular food it can efficiently use that food, no matter what the nutritional level or caloric content that this food would measure in the laboratory. My own experiences, as well as the experiences of others who have followed this method, is that what you feel about yourself and your relationship to the food you are eating has an impact on how that food will be used in your body. I believe that when you crave a food, you should eat it. Cravings are authentic inner signals.

If you crave a chocolate cake, by all means, get one. Declare it a meal and eat it in the regular One Bowl way, by yourself, in your bowl, until you are no longer hungry. If, the next time you feel hungry, that chocolate cake hums again, eat it again in the One Bowl way. Don't worry, you will not eat chocolate cake for the rest of your life and gain a thousand pounds! But eat cake when it hums. Never deprive yourself. Just pay attention to each bite as you have already learned to do. Sooner or later, your craving will lessen or disappear. If you are paying attention to your inner food symphony, you may learn powerful things about yourself through your food cravings.

For example, sometimes when I feel a craving coming on, I just retire for a little while to my favorite eating place and experience that craving. I do not try to satisfy it—I just watch it calling to me from deep within. Usually, if left unmet, after a few minutes that craving will diminish and disappear by itself.

So, you might ask, why did I begin this section by saying, "I believe that when you crave a food, you should eat it. Cravings are authentic inner signals." I do, and they are. People who have denied themselves their cravings, or indulged them, then felt guilty about what they've done, need permission to explore their food cravings. That's the only way to gain power over them. As long as a thing is taboo we will desire it—that's the human condition. So, give yourself permission to indulge all your food cravings using the One Bowl method. It won't take you more than a month to discover what cravings are, and to feel at peace with them.

By exploring your food cravings, interesting realizations emerge. For example, I discovered that after I eat beef, I can expect to have a brief but intense sweet tooth. I don't know why this is, and I suspect it is something unique to me. So long ago I learned to eat a cookie, but then I would feel worried that I might gain weight by eating it. Now, I just find a comfortable spot and "watch" my sweet craving arise, intensify, and then diminish. By following this simple observation process, "sweets after meat" no longer has power over me. There's an old saying: "I never need fear what I understand." This aphorism certainly applies here.

Armed with these two choices—to indulge your cravings or just watch them—you can explore your food cravings to see what might be there. First, make a list of any food cravings you think you might have. Then, write down any discoveries you make about your food cravings in your Journal.

THE BALANCED DIET

Dr. Linus Pauling, who discovered the power of vitamin C for strengthening our resistance to infection, addressed the issue of popular misconceptions about nutrition. Pauling had this to say about the validity of the so-called "balanced diet" approach to human nutrition: "The balanced diets publicized nowadays may not meet the needs of one person in a thousand." And he added, "People shouldn't rely on the minimum daily requirement standards set for vitamins and minerals."

Dr. Roger Williams, a biochemist at the University of Texas and a leading expert on our need for micro-nutrients, added: "Nutritional needs vary with every individual. Too little is known about these variations to decide what is a balanced diet and for whom."

Dr. Pauling responded to the question of whether a certain food or vitamin can be good for one condition and bad for another: "I've heard it said that Vitamin C might be good for colds but bad for kidneys. This is ridiculous. Any nutrient that is good for one part of the body will benefit the entire body."

These men were remarkable for their openness and courage. My experience is that most doctors condemn anything that hasn't been measured in the laboratory. They forget that the laboratory was devised over many centuries as a tool for studying human beings, but that *the primary source*, the reality, *lies in the human being him- or herself*, not in the laboratory. Learn to trust your inner signals. You are the primary source. Your body events are your principal reality.

Think about the liquids you drink in a day. How many are there? Coffee, beer, water, tea, soft drinks, liquor, orange juice. It's a long list. I consider all of them to be foods, and I treat them as foods. When I began the One Bowl method, eating only one food per meal from my bowl, and eating alone, I refrained from drinking liquids with my meal. After all, it seemed logical to me that this would be mixing two foods together.

Now when I want something to drink, that drink becomes a food which I subject to the same One Bowl criteria as all other foods. In other words, when I feel thirsty, I hunt for the drink that hums, even if it turns out to be water. Then I drink alone, one swallow at a time, listening for inner signals about this food I am ingesting. Whenever I feel thirsty, I declare it a meal, and drink. When I no longer feel thirsty, I stop drinking.

Since I can have as many meals in a day as I want, there is no problem. If I feel thirsty during a meal, which sometimes happens, I hunt for just the right drink and make it a course in my meal. I treat water the same as milk, coffee, tea, or any soft drink. All are foods available for the taking. If you doubt that the common liquids you drink act in your digestive system as foods, don't take my word for it, use your One Bowl tools and experiment for yourself!

When I drink, do I first pour the liquid into my bowl? Yes, sometimes I do. This is easier when using some bowls than others. A bowl with a wide lip on it is almost impossible to drink from without it spilling all over me, while Anne Franklin's round bottomed bowls are easy to use. Whether or not I drink from my bowl depends on my mood and which bowl I am using at the time. Actually, I find drinking from my bowl to be fun, so I tend to do it when I'm in a playful mood.

DRINKING

EXERCISE:

The purpose of this exercise is to get in touch with how the liquids you put in your body affect you. For one week eat according to the One Bowl concept but drink freely during all your meals. Then, for the next week consider everything you drink to be a meal. Do not drink while you eat. Subject everything you drink to One Bowl criteria. When you feel thirsty hunt for just the right drink you want. As you drink, listen to your inner signals. I find that eating one food and drinking one food together at a meal has the same effect as eating two foods at that meal: The signals from one blur the signals from the other. What did you discover? Record your discoveries in your Food Awareness Journal.

But you might say, don't the foods you drink digest much faster than the foods you eat? They seem to. But the different foods I eat digest at different rates anyway. I see liquid and solid foods all on a continuum; some digest faster than others but they all vary tremendously in the range of their influence on me. What's important is whether I am satisfied during the drinking, and afterward.

> My snacks were my meals,
> and since I could eat anything I
> wanted at any time that I felt hungry,
> my meals were snacks, too.

SNACKS

A s I continued to work with the One Bowl method, I realized that the distinction between meals and snacks had been completely blurred. My snacks were my meals, and since I could eat anything I wanted at any time that I felt hungry, my meals were snacks, too. No longer were my meals obligations and my snacks rewards, a divisive concept that has allowed the food companies to make fortunes. Now all foods could be fun, or none of them. I had regained control of everything. A candy bar was as good as a carrot, was as good as iced tea, was as good as broccoli.

Eating is designed
to ruin your appetite.

No longer did I worry whether eating some food would ruin my appetite later. Of course it would! *Eating is designed to ruin your appetite.* That's partly why we eat! Now I could eat apple pie or potato chips all day long if I really wanted them. All they had to do was hum. The guilt was gone.

I experienced a tremendous elation when the impact of this discovery finally hit me. Every meal was a snack! Now, I regularly subject fun foods to One Bowl criteria and decide for myself if I want to eat them.

But wait, you might protest, if I allow myself that luxury, I will very likely eat hot dogs or chocolate cake forever. I'll totally destroy my digestive system, get my metabolism completely out of kilter, live from sugar high to sugar high and gain a tremendous amount of weight. Oh? You will? Will you really? Some nutritionists and other authority figures have tried to scare us into believing this, but actual research has proved this wrong.

When children in a controlled experiment were encouraged to select anything they wanted from a wide variety of foods, it's true that at first they ate a lot of candy, cake, and ice cream. But, after awhile, they began to choose more nutritious foods. By the end of the experiment, researchers concluded that even children, if left alone, would eat a normal, pretty balanced diet. No one will eat chocolate cake, or anything else, forever—at least not if they are following the One Bowl method and have learned to listen to their inner signals. Try it and see.

The One Bowl method works because it guides you back, one easy step at a time, to a relationship with your body and mind wherein you become increasingly aware of what your entire organism wants and needs to stay healthy. In the process, you are able to sort out the signals that come mostly from your head or from a craving that has more to do with satisfying an emotional need than it does a nutritional one. Harmony in your inner symphony comes when you stop telling your body what to do and start learning to listen to what your whole organism truly wants.

This exercise is about testing what your body will communicate to you when you feed it nothing but sweets.
Buy or make a wonderful, rich, just-perfect-for-you
chocolate cake (or other sweet of your choice). Now,
for the sake of this experiment, forget your One Bowl
method. Today you are going to eat a big piece of this
chocolate cake whenever you are hungry, regardless
of whether you want cake or not. For breakfast—cake.
For mid-morning snack—cake. For lunch—cake. For
mid-afternoon snack—cake. For dinner—cake. And for
that little snack before retiring—cake again.

How are you doing? Record in your Journal the
changing feelings you experience regarding your
interest in this cake. Write down just how long you continued to eat cake, and what you discovered from this
experiment.

I realize, of course, that there are bingers who may sit down to
eat a single slice of cake and will eat the whole cake instead. If you
have had difficulties like this in the past, don't try this exercise
until you have been following the One Bowl diet for several
months. Then, instead of feeling guilty about what you are going

O
N
E

B
O
W
L

to do, give yourself permission to eat the whole cake in one setting, if that is what you really feel compelled to do. But be sure to do it according to the One Bowl method, being fully aware of your organism's reaction to each bite. Bingers tend to be totally unconscious of what they are eating when they are on a binge, and the One Bowl method will force them to be more aware, and ultimately get in touch with the non-food needs they are seeking to satisfy in this way. If you sometimes binge on food, reread the section entitled Symbolic Hunger.

> In such an environment, unless you
> have the resolve of a saint, it is
> going to be virtually impossible to
> stay focused on your food symphony.

EATING OUT

I have never attempted to eat from my bowl in public, either at a restaurant or at someone else's home. My bowl is a personal possession, and an intimate part of my private eating space. But restaurant eating is almost unavoidable in our society, so I have had to make my peace with it while remaining true to the One Bowl method. How do I do that?

Many restaurants serve portions that are way too large. When I ask waiters why they serve such big portions, and sometimes even use oversized plates to do it on, they tell me that their customers demand more food! People seem to want to gorge themselves these days, as if driven by some primitive survival ritual gone amuck. Perhaps it has something to do with getting one's money's worth. And what's a better measure of that than getting so much food you can't eat it all? When I asked a friend of mine why he ate in these restaurants, he said, "Because I like to know that I can go away just stuffed, if that's what I want to do."

Eating in a restaurant is a highly socialized event. Increasingly, when they eat out, people do so for entertainment as much as for nutrition. Not long ago a business associate told me about a restaurant in L.A. where all the waitresses are buxom and topless. While this is an extreme example, it is indicative of a certain direction that restaurant eating has taken in our country—a place to eat, visit with friends, drink, laugh and carry on in ways one probably couldn't do at home. Even in a fairly reasonable family restaurant the activity can be very high energy, even chaotic, with servers rushing too and fro, dishes clattering, laughter and loud voices in the background. Obviously, in such an environment, unless you have the resolve of a saint, it is going to be virtually impossible to stay focused on your inner symphony. When I eat in a restaurant,

I know that I will have to talk to someone and that I will not be able to hear my inner food signals very well.

The bottom line is that restaurant eating often means overeating, as well as less satisfying eating, and I just go with that from the start, not asking for anything to be different than it usually is. When, for one reason or another I have to eat at a restaurant, I accept these limitations.

I eat out only when a social, work, or family situation calls for it. And whenever I agree to go to a restaurant, I try to have as much fun as I can. I don't worry about how I eat. Because I live the One Bowl method, I am not afraid of restaurant eating.

Armed with my new self-knowledge derived from my One Bowl experiments, restaurants exert little influence over how I eat. Now that I eat more with my whole self than my head, I know that there is always a better eating experience waiting for me at home later, and I take comfort in that. Though this pattern is changing, particularly on the two coasts, restaurant eating is all too often greasy, fatty, salty, and sugary, all served in a noisy and too busy atmosphere. When I can't find a restaurant serving healthy foods in quiet surroundings, I come away from the experience more edgy than relaxed, socially stimulated but physically unsettled, and sometimes with minor symptoms of indigestion. Nevertheless, eating out is a part of contemporary life. Taken altogether, I avoid restaurants when I can but when I can't, I remind myself to listen to the signals from within my own body. And if I am conducting business at the restaurant, and will not be able to pay attention to my food symphony, I just go with the program, knowing that I can return to One Bowl the next meal.

I realize, of course, that there are a rare few restaurants that focus on providing a peaceful and pleasant atmosphere, with a good variety of healthy foods from which to choose. In addition, there are increasing numbers of restaurants and natural food markets that cater to health conscious people with a good variety of carry out foods. If you have such a place near you, you are fortunate indeed. For others living in smaller, less sophisticated communities, it continues to be a challenge. To take care of myself in these situations, I use a number of restaurant survival strategies which I'll share with you. I have found that these will work equally well whether I am in a fast food establishment or a fancy restaurant.

First, I view the menu as my happy hunting ground, and I try to visualize each food listed there. I see it in my mind's eye while asking myself whether that food really hums for me. If I can see pictures of the food on display, so much the better. It is interesting to note, by the way, that in the restaurants in many Asian countries, it is customary to display photos of the food served, either in the menu or prominently on the wall. The reason for this is that most Oriental cooking traditions place a great deal of emphasis on the visual appeal of their food. This custom can be seen in many Japanese, Thai, and Chinese restaurants in this country today. I have found that these pictures can aid me in choosing food by the One Bowl method. But photos or not, I work down through the menu as though it were a shelf in my kitchen.

Second, I stay alert to avoid head eating, because for some reason it is a lot easier for me to eat with my head in a restaurant than it is at home. Usually my head will think, "This restaurant is famous for pizza, so I should eat a pizza," or "This restaurant is famous for vegetarian dishes," without considering whether pizza or a specific vegetarian dish actually hums to me at that moment. This is head eating and whenever I choose a meal on this basis, I overeat.

Third, if I am unable to find food that hums from a menu or from the pictures on the walls, I expand my happy hunting ground to include all the people in the room. I excuse myself from the table and slowly wander around the room, looking at the food other people are eating. I have found this to be an excellent way to find a meal that hums, and usually I will make a quick connection. When the server appears, I simply point to the other person's food, even if it is halfway across the room, and inquire: "What is that they are eating?" It's a little crude, but it works.

Fourth, if I am somewhat familiar with the restaurant, I may choose what I want to eat before opening the menu. This strategy will put me in touch with what hums for me—but it may not be on the menu! In that case, I am back to making my selection by scanning the menu or the food other people are eating.

Fifth, sometimes I follow a restaurant survival strategy developed by my wife, Eugenia. There is a restaurant we go to where the food is good but the helpings are often outrageously large. So Eugenia orders the food that most likely hums for her and at the same time requests that they bring her a take-home box. When her meal arrives, before eating a bite of it, she transfers at least half of everything on her plate into the take-home box, closes the lid, sets it aside and eats her meal. When we have finished eating, she leaves the take-home box on the table. This way, she doesn't overeat, and she doesn't have to eat the same meal again the next day, when no doubt it will no longer hum for her.

Sixth, most dinners in restaurants come with three or four different foods on the same large plate. My tactic for dealing with this un-One Bowl-like situation is to eat from my plate in courses. That is, I will eat the one food on my plate that most hums first, and continue to eat it by itself until I feel satisfied. Then I pause to check in with myself to see if I still feel hungry or to see if one of the other foods on my plate hums. If I can't tell what I am feeling, I sometimes excuse myself, go to the bar, or to the men's room, or even step outside, taking this time to check in with myself.

Seventh, while I am eating, I visualize my bowl. This helps me keep in touch with my inner symphony even though the bowl is sitting in its special place, waiting for me at home. I find that I can usually do this kind of simple visualization while talking or listening to other people. Then, when my hunger ceases, I stop eating and just leave the remaining food on my plate.

But leaving food on your plate challenges convention. It's almost un-American. If someone has taken me out to dinner for a special occasion, they may feel insulted or hurt that I didn't eat everything. Or maybe a server will ask if there was something wrong with the food. A simple, "No, nothing wrong. It was delicious. I just didn't want to overeat," will usually be sufficient to stop any further discussion.

When all else fails, I just let myself overeat, knowing that I can easily repair the damage later. What usually happens is that I have a much smaller appetite than the folks I am eating with, so I will get full pretty quickly. Knowing this, I feel free to chat with them and otherwise let myself be distracted. This makes eating out more enjoyable, because I can focus on it as a social rather than a nutritional event.

> Restaurants mirror the social
> conventions around food in our
> culture—and for the most part, they
> are extraordinarily unhealthy.

I thought about devising an exercise for eating in a restaurant until I realized that restaurant eating itself is the exercise! The exercise is to eat in any restaurant and try to find ways to remain in touch with yourself and your inner symphony of signals while you do so. The next time you eat out, give it a try. Record your discoveries in your Journal.

RESTAURANT EATING

From my own experiences in restaurants, I am faced with one inescapable conclusion: Restaurants mirror our social conventions around food—and for the most part, they are a challenge to anyone following the One Bowl method. Although there are exceptions, I've found that most restaurants lead me away from myself, and they make me overeat usually unhealthy foods. Increasingly I have to make serious choices about what I am going to feed my body and my soul. Just as I have to be conscious of the fact that sitting through a movie where people are being abused and brutally murdered may be entertaining but will have a negative impact on my soul, I also have to become more conscious of how sitting through a meal at a noisy, chaotic restaurant will have a negative impact on my body. My first choice is always to avoid those situations where I know the eating experience is going to have a negative impact on me.

Recently, there has been, in the west and in the southern states, a rise in the popularity of cafeterias that serve a wide variety of foods, among which are some very healthy ones. These are the only form of restaurants I know of where it is possible to hunt your own food and satisfy yourself without over-eating. You glide your tray down the rails in front of the food windows through which you can see a wide selection of salads, meats, vegetables, breads, desserts, and drinks. It is easy to hunt for just the right food. The servings are small, each single food item comes in its own dish, but you pay for all-you-can-eat, so you can consider the entire cafeteria your happy hunting ground.

Today I ate lunch by myself at Furr's Cafeteria, an old Texas chain that has spread west to California. I had chosen a salad and was hunting for a possible meat dish. But nothing hummed. Then I spotted the fried fish and was about to order a serving when I felt a slight weight in my stomach—just a small sensation, forecasting how my stomach would feel if I ate the fish. So I passed on it and passed on the meats entirely. Then I found two vegetables and mashed potatoes. These hummed. I had a great meal. To my mind, a good cafeteria is about as close to eating out One Bowl–style as I can imagine. If you have a cafeteria near you, give it a try.

Eating at someone else's home is better still. I usually feel I have more control there because I feel freer to choose the amount of food I will eat. If asked why I am not taking seconds, I usually explain by saying, "I am a light eater." This comment will satisfy almost everyone except mothers-in-law. It also prevents me from getting into that spot where I have to choose between overeating or hurting someone's feelings. And invariably someone at the table turns out to be very interested in new food and diet ideas, and if I mention One Bowl, usually a good conversation follows.

GUILT AND WEIGHT-CONSCIOUSNESS

In writing this book it is impossible to ignore the fact that any time eating is discussed it invariably is seen as a weight issue. Losing weight and conforming to current fashionable body measurements is after all an 11-billion-dollar-a-year industry. Body size and fitness have become something akin to a contemporary morality. Not conforming is akin to being a sin. People on weight-loss diets often feel guilty, as if being overweight is evil, as if they have done something wrong and dieting is their penance. They feel guilty no matter which way they go; if they don't diet they feel bad about being fat. If they diet they feel bad about having to endure their cruel penance. The result is that they have no power over food in their lives, and cannot really enjoy eating. This leads to the feast or famine phenomenon, which means either overeating or strict dieting. The One Bowl method can stop this yo-yoing dilemma forever, turning true food awareness into a philosophy of life, something that guides us in discovering more about ourselves and the bigger picture of life. Awareness of my eating thus becomes a source of pride and high self-esteem, something I eagerly share with everybody.

I have found in the past twenty-plus years of following this eating method that many people like to talk about the meaning of food in their lives when they realize that they can talk to me openly, and because I have an unusual approach. Try talking about your One Bowl experiences with your friends. It may make social eating more meaningful. . . . and healthier for you.

CARRY FOOD WITH YOU

I have learned one other thing that I want to pass along to you. I usually carry a little food with me when I am away from my living space. I know that every three or four hours I must eat to keep my energy even and constant, so I prepare for that. When I attend business conferences, I either find a time when it's all right to eat the food I've brought, or I excuse myself and go eat privately. There is no reason to ignore my body signals of hunger just because I am in a social situation. I use my creativity to carve out a good food space for myself. I sometimes say I need to visit the bathroom, then I step outside for a snack instead. I sometimes use prepackaged energy bars for this because they don't melt or spoil so easily. Other times I carry hard-boiled eggs, carrot sticks, and finger foods that won't spoil during the time I am away.

Once I had learned how to understand my inner food signals, I found that they operated every day regardless of social customs. In order to make the One Bowl method work, I found that I had to follow it regularly. But more profoundly, I found that I wanted to follow it regularly. Pretty soon I preferred feeling good and having a steady energy flow throughout the day. I chose to live that way rather than falling back into the old patterns that rewarded me with erratic sensations of hunger and fullness. That realization made it really important for me to stay with my inner food feelings, no matter what the social situation happened to be. As you become more comfortable with One Bowl eating, the same can happen for you and you will automatically use your creativity to find ways to maintain your chosen food habits regardless of the social situation.

I recently read that the average city dweller in the U.S. now eats at least four restaurant meals per week, and many thousands of Americans eat most of their meals out. This means that the majority of people in our culture almost always eat in environments where they have limited food selections and little or no control over noise levels, physical activity, or prevailing (usually chaotic) atmosphere.

Besides restaurant eating, where we may have a very limited hunting ground in most areas of the country, millions of people rarely prepare food for themselves. At best, a spouse or one other family member selects the menus and prepares the food. This practice is a more subtle form of food socialization than eating with other people, since it means you eat food dominated by the mood, or the desires, or the economics of another person. The person preparing the food may be serving what hums for them— but not necessarily what hums for you. Or worse, that person may

ONE BOWL

be trying to please you—to anticipate the food you would like—so that the food you eat rarely fits anyone's needs, yours or theirs.

It seems that everyone has silently agreed to eat within a certain narrow range or selection of food. This is the process by which families commonly build up their eating patterns, which usually come down to everyone eating things that the food provider likes or thinks they should have. This may mean that most of the time nobody is happy. What's worse, this system teaches us that there is nothing we can do about our food choices, regardless of what our insides are telling us, so we might as well just "eat what's put in front of you."

When you start eating the One Bowl way, you liberate yourself from the double-binds you've been accepting as a fact of life until now. Although well-meaning, family eating patterns can certainly turn into a kind of food tyranny that I firmly believe is the foundation of most of our eating disorders in this country. According to the Surgeon General, obesity is epidemic in America! And remember, obesity is simply the most obvious symptom of being out touch with the inner signals of our bodies.

After giving it some thought, I realized that in my own family structure at least, I could break free to make my own food choices if I was willing to prepare my food myself. Although getting free required a number of discussions and explanations with my wife and the kids, once I did so a new world opened up before me and food preparation, preceded by food hunting, became a new and important adventure for me.

At first, my family's primary food provider, Eugenia, thought my new ideas meant that I didn't love her anymore. And she didn't appreciate my labeling her cooking as food tyranny! It took me a few days to convince her that I meant this in a conceptual, not a personal, sense. Although she had slaved for years as our food provider, she did not want to give it up. She had trouble surrendering that role to a new system in which each of us cooked for him or her self. But in time, we evolve a new method. We learned to cook for ourselves together. Try it. It's fun.

> The most important ingredient in
> food preparation is my mood.

FOOD PREPARATION

The most important ingredient in food preparation is my mood. I like to be hungry but in a carefree state, physically and emotionally relaxed, when I begin to prepare my food. If I have chosen it well, getting just the right food to eat, I want to prepare it lovingly and creatively. Usually I begin by imagining how I will prepare it. This mental projection can be just an instant flash or it can take several moments of elaborate contemplation. This allows me to test out what I want to do with my food before I eat it. Sometimes I want to dream or fantasize about it; sometimes I want to caress or fondle it. Sometimes I play with it. Sometimes I conquer it. Occasionally, I am just efficient and businesslike in my preparation of it. All of these moods and many more are a necessary part of eating to me now. When I allow myself to express my mood in food preparation, it whets my appetite and also satisfies something deep within.

In such a mood I really look at the food I am preparing and I really touch it. I wash it and cut it while I think about washing it and cutting it. My attention is on the food because I am really interested in it. It hums, and I really want to eat it.

Usually by the time I am ready to eat it I know my food pretty well. To me food preparation means preparing both the food and my organism for the coming transformation we will both undergo by my eating it. This food I hold in my hands will soon become a part of me. I have to ready myself to receive it. The food will be changed by my eating; but equally important, *I will be changed by the food.*

I was recently visiting in a friend's home when they gave the family dog a new bone. The dog wagged its tail excitedly, parading past me with the bone in her mouth. She then settled down in the corner of the room that she identified as her special place. I watched in amazement as she placed the bone on the floor and rolled over on top of it. She seemed to deeply enjoy this process, rubbing her back, her cheeks, and her ears against this wonderful bone she'd just received. It was as if she was blending herself—her own scents and the oils from her fur—with the scents and oils of her wonderful new prize. Only after doing this for several minutes did she at last hold the bone between her paws and start gnawing on it, sheer ecstasy lighting up her face. She was indeed in Doggy Heaven!

As I watched I couldn't help but compare this dog's rituals of preparation to the spirit of food preparation that I enjoy in my life. If we are paying attention in the One Bowl way, food preparation becomes much more than chopping, heating and stirring. Like the dog with her new bone, we are literally mingling our own energies with the food prior to taking full possession of it by chewing it up and incorporating it into our being.

I have a friend whose wife always has a wonderful, lush kitchen garden in a small raised plot on their city lot. She grows beautiful tomatoes, zucchini, bell peppers, lettuce, and onions. In the middle of the summer there are fresh strawberries from earthen strawberry pots that she lovingly cultivates. In the winter there are

ONE BOWL

crops such as broccoli and mustard greens. As evening approaches, husband and wife are often found in the garden, choosing what they will prepare for their meal that night. The whole process, from growing to harvesting to preparation and finally eating is very hands-on and conscious, and this couple loves each step in the process, from cultivating the soil through eating the fruits of their labor.

While we don't all have the ability to live as my friends do, they remind us both of what's possible and of the intimate relationship we historically have had with our food, a relationship that is virtually lost in contemporary life. However, I believe that through the One Bowl method we can recapture much of this experience, whether we are living in a high rise in New York City or on a thousand-acre ranch in Iowa.

SEASONINGS

I have learned to season my foods with small amounts of other foods, which is what commercial seasonings are anyway. The only difference is that mine are always fresh. Among my favorite seasonings are celery, pecans, walnuts, cheese, mushrooms, onions, occasionally garlic, parsley, olives, and radishes. Each of these seasonings was subjected to One Bowl criteria; each evolved into my hunting ground over a period of months. Like all the other foods I eat, the seasonings I use slowly change as I grow and change.

Seasonings are of course just a small amount of another food, so eating any seasoning on your food is like eating two or three foods together. The resultant new food I create in this way, I subject to all of my One Bowl criteria. If the new food is harmonious to my body, then it stays in my happy hunting ground and I use it when it hums.

TASSAJARA COOKING

About the time I refined the One Bowl method of eating to its present state, I discovered a wonderful book, entitled *The Tassajara Cookbook*. This book is now out of print but by using the Internet it may be possible to find used copies of it through used book websites such as www.Bookfinders.com. *The Tassajara Cookbook* devotes loving attention to food preparation, showing how to focus on a single food at a time. It showed me how to get to know a food as I prepared it and it gave me many new food preparation ideas. The book has no regular recipes to follow but it did help me invent some for myself. I found that by reading it like a story I could take many imaginary food preparation adventures. You might enjoy it too, and I consider it a welcome complement to the One Bowl method.

Going further physically means expanding the attention you focus on your digestive system to include your mouth and teeth, and your bowels. If you find that getting in touch with your body functions through the concepts presented here is meaningful to you, then you may be interested in trying these explorations.

TEETH

The way I explore my teeth is simple. I am interested in learning what my teeth feel like before and after I eat, and in how my bowels function to excrete waste. Teeth and bowels are not exactly socially popular subjects in our culture. But because self-knowledge and body health go together, I decided to explore these taboo areas.

If I try to describe what my teeth feel like, I find it difficult to do. But after brushing them well, then flossing, I know that they feel different than before I cleaned them. After a meal, I sit for a minute and feel my teeth. They definitely are different now, a new

ONE BOWL

feeling. Any time I run my tongue over them I can feel where there are food-covered surfaces and little patches of food. Eating different foods leaves me with different tooth-surface sensations.

Gradually, over a year of exploration, I found that I preferred the way my teeth felt when they were clean. So after I eat, I usually do this: First, I run my tongue over all the surfaces, cleaning off the food. Then I use water to rinse my mouth. These things I can do even when eating out—I just excuse myself and go to the restroom. Next, at the first chance I get, I brush. I find it easy to carry a folding travel toothbrush in my pocket everywhere I go. In public, there's always a restroom available.

Not everyone might want to brush as often as I do. My wife, Eugenia, prefers to leave the taste of a good meal in her mouth for as long as possible. You might too, and if so, do it.

I learned from Dr. Thomas McGuire's *Tooth Fitness* how to brush and floss to prevent cavities. I learned to tell by the feel of my tongue and the taste in my mouth when my teeth were dirty. I learned to brush part of the time without toothpaste because its taste confused my ability to tell when my teeth really were clean. I also learned from his book that contrary to a lot of expensive advertising, bad breath is caused by poor eating and lousy digestive habits. Using the One Bowl method allowed me to give up mouthwash.

I have been exploring food awareness in my life for more than twenty-six years now. *Tooth Fitness* is an excellent primer on food and diet. Dr. Thomas McGuire modernizes the pioneering work begun in his classic book, *The Tooth Trip* (which I had the honor to publish in 1972 but which is now long out of print). *Tooth Fitness, Your Guide To Healthy Teeth*, updates Thomas' work in *The Tooth Trip* and is a must have. *Tooth Fitness* is available from Amazon.com, or any general bookstore.

ELIMINATION

I understand the basic movement of biological life to be a two-part process. The body gathers to itself new possessions and eliminates from itself used materials or materials it no longer needs. This movement has been described as charge and discharge, or as "transposition." However you view it, we are talking about the fundamental biological rhythm of life. The American culture has been characterized as one in which people easily add possessions, but give them up only with difficulty. We fill our homes, then our garages, and when our garages are full we rent storage spaces. This practice may explain why we consider elimination and the organs of elimination taboo. I sometimes get the image of people grown fat because they eat but don't eliminate.

ONE BOWL

They prefer to store food up within themselves rather than surrender it back to the world.

My point is that elimination is just as important as eating, but it is not given proper attention. Many people solve the elimination problem by taking laxatives, but they are not good for you and also force the body to do what it prefers to do naturally.

I explored my inner signals about elimination in this way: Each morning I lay on the floor with my knees up and the bottoms of my feet flat on the floor. I tried to focus my attention on my intestines just inside my anus and waited to feel movement there. For many mornings nothing happened. Sometimes I imagined I felt the movement. Sometimes I grew irritated with myself for wasting time in this way. Other times I tried to be more patient.

When I actually defecated, I would never push. My method was to get in touch with the natural intestinal movements of my body and to see whether I could stimulate them. After almost a year of this I began making progress in contacting this inner movement. Today it has become second nature to me and an integral part of the One Bowl process. I have found that changes in my diet, through One Bowl criteria, have resulted in a new, freer elimination pattern that gives me added assurance about the health of my digestive system. I have found that elimination never requires pushing or straining and that giving it this caring attention helps to maintain this important body function in a healthy state. I definitely spend less time and energy worrying about elimination now than I did before developing the One Bowl method, and I feel that the work I have done has been well repaid. I never have to use laxatives, antacids, or any other drugs or medical remedies.

The only book I know of which can help you with this exploration is *Breathe Away Your Tension,* by Dr. Bruno Geba. The book is now out of print but you might be able to get a copy from www.Bookfinders.com.

> You can begin to apply the tools of
> understanding and exploration you
> have learned in this book to other
> parts of your body and your being.

GOING FURTHER

Once you have expanded your attention into these new areas of your life, you will see that the paths to health and self-knowledge are intertwined. But there is more; you can go further still. For one thing, you can begin to apply the tools of understanding and exploration you have learned in this book to other

ONE BOWL

parts of your body and your being. In this section I will describe a series of very good books, each of which will lead you further down the path to self-awareness. When choosing among them, start with the one that hums (of course!).

To build a firm foundation, I suggest you read some of the classic books by Stanley Keleman, who may be America's greatest philosopher of the body. I strongly recommend both *The Human Ground* and *Living Your Dying* as a great way to expand your growing self-awareness. They will set you on the path to true embodiment. Dr. Keleman's books can be ordered from The Center Press, 2045 Francisco Street, Berkeley, CA 94709. These books, which are published in limited editions, are so insightful and informative that they shouldn't be missed.

Massage for Total Well-Being, by Anne Kent Rush—a woman who pioneered massage in America in the 1970s—is a book which tells how to use acupressure points for body awareness and exploration. One of the prominent acupressure centers is the stomach, so this book can be valuable to your food explorations. Kent has also written *The Modern Book of Massage*, which helps you use acupressure massage to reduce tension and stress. Both of these books are available from Amazon.com, or any general bookstore.

TriEnergetics, by Sanford Severin, M.D. and Todd Severin, M.D. is a new, powerful, comprehensive, unique and fact-filled medical book which will guide you in integrating food awareness, breathing, and physical fitness within a congruent Taoist philosophy. *TriEnergetics* comes highly recommended and is available from Amazon.com, or any general bookstore.

The Well Body Book, by Mike Samuels, M.D. and Hal Zina Bennett is the original, classic alternative home health handbook. Its extraordinary techniques, developed in the 1970s, are still valid today. You might be able to find this book on www.Bookfinders.com, but even used copies are rare because most people won't part with them. At the time of this writing, I discovered six different used book dealers (through Bookfinders.com) who are asking $35 for a used copy in moderately good condition. That's a lot of money for a book that originally sold for $5.95 but still well worth it for anyone who is serious about pursuing these methods of self-exploration for health.

Energy Healing: A Pathway to Inner Growth, by Jim Gilkeson, tells how to explore energy within your own body. His "Etheric Laboratory" sections are excellent, providing a balance between intellectual information and self-exploration exercises. In the first laboratory there's a chapter titled "Trusting the Authority of Your Own

Experience," which is particularly relevant if you are interested in pursuing the One Bowl ideas further. Like *One Bowl*, *Energy Healing* is published by Avalon.

Healing With Love, by Leonard Laskow, M.D., explores how energy, breath, and love contribute to our overall health and sense of well-being. Deepak Chopra, M.D. says of this book, "It offers practical insight into the mechanics of restoration of wholeness. I highly recommend it." Widely available in bookstores or order through that author's website, which is: www.laskow.net

Deep Healing: The Essence of Mind/Body Medicine, by Emmett E. Miller, M.D., is filled with "Experiential Workouts," including checklists, relaxation exercises, mental visualizations, and affirmations to explore the self-healing mechanisms that we all inherit at birth. Most valuable for its contribution to creating wellness through increased self awareness, its focus is self-knowledge and maintaining an optimal experience of health in your everyday life. Widely available.

Spirit Animals and the Wheel of Life: A Nature-Based Spiritual Practice for Everyday Life by Hal Zina Bennett draws from ancient shamanic practices, such as medicine wheel teachings and using animals as teachers, to examine ways to live more fully as a complete, congruent organism, connected with the living forces we call our "environment." This book's "ecospiritual" approach is in full alignment with the One Bowl idea, applied to a deepening understanding of how our own choices and actions have an impact on other people around us as well as on the very Earth under our feet, upon when we are totally dependent. Widely available.

> You can begin by wanting to lose a
> few pounds and end up transforming
> your basic ways of being in the world.

REACHING THE FRONTIER

If by following the simple method set forth in this book, you have carried your self-understanding to this point, you are reaching toward the frontiers of this work. Preventive medicine— or more accurately "wellness medicine"—is a rediscovered, expanding field, devoted to physical and psychic self-exploration. I have mentioned the above books because they can be stepping stones along your path. Most people I know who begin to understand how to make natural changes in their diet want to go beyond their original goal. You can begin by wanting to lose a few pounds and end up transforming your basic ways of being in the world.

USING YOUR FOOD AWARENESS JOURNAL

If you have kept a Food Awareness Journal of your One Bowl discoveries, by this point that book will contain a great deal of valuable information about you. It might be appropriate to consign your Food Awareness Journal to the bookshelves as a valuable record of this work, or even share it with a friend. If, on the other hand you choose to continue your investigations into food awareness, or body awareness, be sure to continue to record these discoveries as well.

In any case, before you put your Journal away, consider taking a quiet hour or two to read back over your past entries. If you dated your exercises and explorations each time you made an entry, you will be able to trace how your understanding and awareness grew. Many people get new insights from retracing the path they have taken. I hope you will, too.

PEACE OF MIND

I began this quest because I wanted to lose twenty pounds but that quest took me along a path of more complete self-awareness

ONE BOWL

167

that continues even to this day. The time I spent sitting, taking a bite of food every few minutes, and listening to the food symphony playing inside of me, led me to explore paths I had never imagined existed when I began. For one thing, it led me to write this book. For another, it led me to discover how to be much more content with myself. This is a direct result of simply wanting to focus on the food energy inside me, but it has brought another world into view. I now see that the path which opened up to me on this journey didn't stop with food awareness. It expanded out to embrace every aspect of my life.

One Bowl has carried me into a personal way of being that is more peaceful, that allows me to detach myself from my cares, and experience myself as a whole organism, a living, connected being, congruent, without name or desire. This is a state in which I do not know myself by thinking and do not talk to myself with words. It is a silent state, a state of pure sensation; it has no boundaries. Within it I am no longer a mind and a body with a name, I am pure being. And I am content. I have become my body. I am it and it is me.

Body sensations are my language. I live life slowly, at what I imagine to be a biochemical rate of speed. Most of the time I feel immensely calm and secure. I value this state in my life enough to try to enter it at least once a day.

ONE BOWL

Down through history people have discovered this state for themselves and have called it by many names—prayer, meditation, enlightenment, and Being-At-One, are a few of them. You can use the knowledge you have learned by practicing the One Bowl method to begin to open yourself to this congruent inner experience, too.

I get into this special state the same way that I listen to food messages, except that now I listen for messages anywhere in my entire being, but not of course when I'm eating. I just listen for whatever is occurring within. I focus my attention first on the sensations of:

> the pulsation of my heartbeat
> the rhythm of my breathing

I relax any tense muscles I feel. My breathing slows and I feel my breath fall lower into my abdomen. I just let it go. After a few moments of this, I pay attention to sensations of

> falling
> tingling
> changes in weight, pressure, temperature
> emptiness

Soon it is just as though a door has closed, shutting out the world. I am internally quiet, sometimes floating, at peace.

At first these feelings made me uneasy because they were quite unfamiliar. When I tried to evaluate them or interpret them I had difficulty keeping them in focus. One day I realized that all of these sensations, even the strangest ones, were me. After that, I found it easier to explore them. Now I am learning how to travel around among the sensations in my being, and throughout its many parts. The more I follow this path, the more I secure for myself an inner sanctuary against the storm of desires and ambitions that fill the world. This brings me a continual peace.

If you are a person who enjoys being with yourself, you may enjoy this state. Any time you feel tense or hyperactive, you can find relaxation and well-being here. In college, I read a wonderful book entitled *The Sound Of Silence*. The book stated that all sound is merely vibration, and as such, is not continuous. It is a series of short noise bursts separated by instants of silence. The book advised me, if I wanted to find peace, to listen to the silence between the sounds.

Douglas Harding has described this same idea using the visual medium in his extraordinary book entitled *On Having No Head*. If either of these ideas hum for you, by all means "eat" them.

A good philosophical work that will bring you to this same conclusion from the tradition of Christian Theology, is Soren Kierkegaard's *Purity of Heart Is to Will One Thing*. Or, if you want to explore a different way, you might want to read Sri Nissargadatta Maharaj's powerful *I Am That*. These books are available from Amazon.com, or any general bookstore.

CREATING YOURSELF

I developed One Bowl by using my common sense and by trusting my belief that the feelings I experienced inside of me were real and valid, and were important to my well-being. I also believed that my body contained its own inner wisdom which, with diligent effort, I could learn to heed. I also believed that my body had the ability to choose how to be healthy. Given half a chance, it would always act in the most healthy way it could.

Over time I discovered that these beliefs really worked, and this experience was the foundation from which the One Bowl method evolved. Good feelings about the role of food in my life also helped me rely more and more on my own power to care for myself.

The ideas presented in this book rest firmly on my experiences; they are reaffirmed and renewed continually in my daily life.

ONE BOWL

Human experience is passed on and can be verified by others. Do not take my word for it but experiment for yourself. A new world awaits. Through this book I am passing my experience to you.

ATTAINING CONGRUENCY

More than two decades have passed since I began exploring the basic principles of food awareness that fill this book and the method has gone through many tests and many changes. Soon after starting this work, I discovered European constitutional homeopathy, a form of Western medicine that has built its therapeutics on the uniqueness of human individuality, not on a computer model of common symptoms. Here was a medical system that shared the same principles as the One Bowl method!

I soon gave this form of homeopathy a try. To my surprise, it really worked. I began to go much further. My inner experience soon became a path for deep constitutional healing as well. The One Bowl method was not only completely compatible with the homeopathic work, it became fully integrated with it almost immediately. Since that time, I have used European constitutional homeopathy continuously without taking any allopathic (American medical) drugs—not even so much as an aspirin.

I share this story because I know that as you follow the One

ONE BOWL

172

Bowl method you may find your understanding and your beliefs changing. In the process you may find yourself in conflict with beliefs and systems that you once accepted or even cherished. At such times you may find yourself feeling that you have to choose between one set of beliefs and another. But there is another way, and that is to seek further. If your new experiences have fostered new beliefs, look for what is compatible with those beliefs, even if it means searching far afield and challenging what you held to be true in the past. For me that search led me to European constitutional homeopathy. For you the path may lead elsewhere. Apply the One Bowl method even here, and you'll do fine. Just as with choosing the food that hums for you, you'll find what's right for you by choosing the way of life that hums for you.

As the years pass, I experience an increased congruence in my life, more energy, and far fewer symptoms of illness than I have ever known. European constitutional homeopathy, along with the One Bowl method, have together brought a deep inner peace which I would like to give to everybody.

VISIT THE ONE BOWL WEBSITE

If you cannot find a round-bottomed bowl, but you have Internet capability, visit the One Bowl website. The One Bowl internet address is www.onebowlbook.com. Be sure you type the "book" part in. (If you type in simply www.onebowl.com, you will get Kraft Foods.)

At my One Bowl website I feature the beautiful and unique, hand-made, round-bottomed bowls of artist Anne Franklin. Anne has created a line of ceramic, round-bottomed bowls especially for use with the One Bowl method. These bowls each hold between one and one and a half cups of food, just the right amount. In addition, they are powerful spiritual objects in their own right, and they are moderately priced. No two bowls are exactly alike. And they feel great in your hand.

You can choose from a variety of Earth colors, order your bowl right from our website, and pay with your credit card. We try to ship every order within three days so that you can start using your new bowl as soon as possible.

Trust yourself to live your own journey!

ONE BOWL

www.onebowlbook.com